Obstetric Emergencies

Editor

JAMES M. ALEXANDER

OBSTETRICS AND GYNECOLOGY CLINICS OF NORTH AMERICA

www.obgyn.theclinics.com

Consulting Editor
WILLIAM F. RAYBURN

March 2013 • Volume 40 • Number 1

ELSEVIER

1600 John F. Kennedy Boulevard • Suite 1800 • Philadelphia, Pennsylvania, 19103-2899

http://www.theclinics.com

OBSTETRICS AND GYNECOLOGY CLINICS OF NORTH AMERICA Volume 40, Number 1
March 2013 ISSN 0889-8545, ISBN-13: 978-1-4557-7127-1

Editor: Stephanie Donley

Obstetrics and Gynecology Clinics (ISSN 0889-8545) is published quarterly by Elsevier Inc., 360 Park Avenue South, New York, NY 10010-1710. Months of issue are March, June, September, and December. Periodicals postage paid at New York, NY, and additional mailing offices. Subscription price per year is $293.00 (US individuals), $518.00 (US institutions), $146.00 (US students), $353.00 (Canadian individuals), $652.00 (Canadian institutions), $214.00 (Canadian students), $428.00 (foreign individuals), $652.00 (foreign institutions), and $214.00 (foreign students). To receive student/resident rate, orders must be accompanied by name of affiliated institution, date of term, and the signature of program/residency coordinator on institution letterhead. Orders will be billed at individual rate until proof of status is received. Foreign air speed delivery is included in all *Clinics* subscription prices. All prices are subject to change without notice. POSTMASTER: Send address changes to *Obstetrics and Gynecology Clinics*, Elsevier Health Sciences Division, Subscription Customer Service, 3251 Riverport Lane, Maryland Heights, MO 63043. **Customer Service: Telephone: 1-800-654-2452 (U.S. and Canada); 314-447-8871 (outside U.S. and Canada). Fax: 314-447-8029. E-mail: journalscustomerservice-usa@elsevier.com (for print support); journalsonlinesupport-usa@elsevier.com (for online support).**

Reprints. For copies of 100 or more of articles in this publication, please contact the Commercial Reprints Department, Elsevier Inc., 360 Park Avenue South, New York, New York 10010-1710. Tel.: 212-633-3818; Fax: 212-462-1935; E-mail: reprints@elsevier.com.

Obstetrics and Gynecology Clinics of North America is also published in Spanish by McGraw-Hill Interamericana Editores S.A., P.O. Box 5-237, 06500, Mexico; in Portuguese by Reichmann and Affonso Editores, Rio de Janeiro, Brazil; and in Greek by Paschalidis Medical Publications, Athens, Greece.

Obstetrics and Gynecology Clinics of North America is covered in MEDLINE/PubMed (Index Medicus), Excerpta Medica, Current Concepts/Clinical Medicine, Science Citation Index, BIOSIS, CINAHL, and ISI/BIOMED.

Printed and bound by CPI Group (UK) Ltd, Croydon, CR0 4YY

Transferred to Digital Printing, 2013

Contributors

CONSULTING EDITOR

WILLIAM F. RAYBURN, MD, MBA
Randolph Seligman Professor and Chair, Department of Obstetrics and Gynecology, University of New Mexico School of Medicine, Albuquerque, New Mexico

EDITOR

JAMES M. ALEXANDER, MD
Chief of Obstetrics, Parkland Hospital; Professor, Department of Obstetrics and Gynecology, Division of Maternal Fetal Medicine; Vice Chairman, Institutional Review Board, University of Texas Southwestern Medical Center, Dallas, Texas

AUTHORS

JAMES M. ALEXANDER, MD
Chief of Obstetrics, Parkland Hospital; Professor, Department of Obstetrics and Gynecology, Division of Maternal Fetal Medicine; Vice Chairman, Institutional Review Board, University of Texas Southwestern Medical Center, Dallas, Texas

MATTHEW C. BRENNAN, MD
Division of Maternal Fetal Medicine, Department of Obstetrics and Gynecology, School of Medicine, University of New Mexico, Albuquerque, New Mexico

STEFFEN BROWN, MD
Fellow and Visiting Instructor, Division of Maternal Fetal Medicine, Department of Obstetrics and Gynecology, University of New Mexico School of Medicine, Albuquerque, New Mexico

CHRISTOPHER GOODIER, MD
Instructor, Medical University of South Carolina, Charleston, South Carolina

WILLIAM GROBMAN, MD, MBA
Professor, Department of Obstetrics and Gynecology, Feinberg School of Medicine, Northwestern University, Chicago, Illinois

BRADLEY D. HOLBROOK, MD
Resident Physician, Department of Obstetrics and Gynecology, University of New Mexico School of Medicine, Albuquerque, New Mexico

LISA E. MOORE, MD
Division of Maternal Fetal Medicine, Department of Obstetrics and Gynecology, School of Medicine, University of New Mexico, Albuquerque, New Mexico

JAMIE MORGAN, MD
Fellow, Maternal-Fetal Medicine, University of Texas Southwestern Medical Center, Texas

ELLEN MOZURKEWICH, MD, MS
Associate Professor, Division of Maternal Fetal Medicine, Department of Obstetrics and Gynecology, University of New Mexico School of Medicine, Albuquerque, New Mexico

SHARON T. PHELAN, MD
Professor, Department of Obstetrics and Gynecology, University of New Mexico School of Medicine, Albuquerque, New Mexico

WILLIAM F. RAYBURN, MD, MBA
Randolph Seligman Professor and Chair, Department of Obstetrics and Gynecology, University of New Mexico School of Medicine, Albuquerque, New Mexico

SCOTT ROBERTS, MD, MSc
Professor, Obstetrics and Gynecology, Maternal-Fetal Medicine, University of Texas Southwestern Medical Center, Dallas, Texas

SCOTT A. SULLIVAN, MD, MSCR
Associate Professor and Director of Maternal Fetal Medicine, Medical University of South Carolina, Charleston, South Carolina

JOEY E. TYNER, MD
Division of Maternal Fetal Medicine, Department of Obstetrics and Gynecology, University of New Mexico School of Medicine, Albuquerque, New Mexico

KAREN L. WILSON, MD, FACOG
Fellow, Department of Obstetrics and Gynecology, University of Texas Southwestern Medical Center, Dallas, Texas

ALISON C. WORTMAN, MD
Fellow, Department of Obstetrics and Gynecology, University of Texas Southwestern Medical Center, Dallas, Texas

Contents

> Umbilical cord prolapse is an obstetric emergency that can have negative outcomes for the fetus. It is diagnosed by a palpable or visible cord and is often accompanied by severe, rapid fetal heart rate decelerations. Cases of cord prolapse should be delivered as soon as possible, usually by cesarean section. While awaiting delivery, the fetal presenting part should be elevated off the cord either manually or by filling the bladder. Although an untreated case of umbilical cord prolapse can lead to severe fetal morbidity and mortality, prompt and appropriate management leads to good overall outcomes.

> Intrapartum hemorrhage is a serious and sometimes life-threatening event. Several etiologies are known and include placental abruption, uterine atony, placenta accreta, and genital tract lacerations. Prompt recognition of blood loss, identification of the source of the hemorrhage, volume resuscitation, including red blood cells and blood products when required, will result in excellent maternal outcomes.

> Amniotic fluid embolism and pulmonary embolism are 2 of the most common causes of maternal mortality in the developed world. Symptoms of pulmonary embolism include tachycardia, tachypnea, and shortness of breath, all of which are common complaints in pregnancy. Heightened awareness leads to rapid diagnosis and institution of therapy. Amniotic fluid embolism is associated with maternal collapse. There are currently no proven therapies, although rapid initiation of supportive care may decrease the risk of mortality.

> An emergent cesarean delivery is performed to immediately intervene to improve maternal or fetal outcome for such indications as fetal distress, prolapsed cord, maternal hemorrhage from previa or trauma, uterine rupture, and complete placental abruption. It is paramount to reduce morbidity and mortality by preparing health care providers for special precautions.

and medical management in pregnancy for seizures and intracranial hemorrhage, and how the two can overlap into preeclampsia or eclampsia. This article also highlights some challenging management issues from the obstetrician's perspective.

Scott A. Sullivan and Christopher Goodier

Several potentially fatal endocrine emergencies in relation to obstetrics and gynecology are discussed in the article. Rates of case fatality vary in different series, but range from 10% to 30%. Rapid recognition, prompt supportive care, and intervention likely maximize maternal and fetal outcomes.

Alison C. Wortman and James M. Alexander

Placenta accreta is an abnormal adherence of the placenta to the uterine wall that can lead to significant maternal morbidity and mortality. The incidence of placenta accreta has increased 13-fold since the early 1900s and directly correlates with the increasing cesarean delivery rate. The prenatal diagnosis of placenta accreta by ultrasound along with risk factors including placenta previa and prior cesarean delivery can aid in delivery planning and improved outcomes. Referral to a tertiary care center and the use of a multidisciplinary care team is recommended.

OBSTETRICS AND GYNECOLOGY CLINICS

Foreword

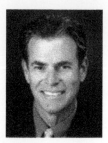

William F. Rayburn, MD, MBA
Consulting Editor

This issue of the *Obstetrics and Gynecology Clinics of North America*, guest edited by Dr James Alexander, represents a contemporary resource on obstetrics in emergent conditions to all individuals in training as well as already established obstetricians. Topics include virtually every condition in obstetrics that requires emergent attention in the Labor and Delivery Unit. The primary goal was to provide the scientific rationale and basis for the procedures rather than to describe the surgical procedures and maneuvers in sufficient detail to serve as a self-instructional text. In doing so, we hoped that the reader would understand why as well as how to regarding these various procedures.

After constructing a comprehensive table of contents, individuals were identified with notable expertise in the various areas to solicit their participation in the project. Each senior contributor not only has extensive experience but also was actively practicing the techniques and surgical procedures described in this issue. Each submission was reviewed to present a consensus perspective of sound clinical judgment.

When more than 1 therapeutic option was valid, the authors attempted to present them all rather than focusing on the preferred technique of the authors. Since many of the described procedures are performed with the aid of anesthesia, attention was placed on each article about obstetric anesthesiology. Simulations available for training or retaining are also discussed in each article.

We hope that this issue will serve as a clinically useful reference for periodic review, either after or preferably before emergencies are encountered. Patient safety is paramount in the field of operative obstetrics, and it is hoped that this issue will provide both practical and timely information to reduce risk. I would like to acknowledge all the authors whose efforts and work helped lay the framework and foundation for this comprehensive text.

William F. Rayburn, MD, MBA
Department of Obstetrics and Gynecology
University of New Mexico School of Medicine
MSC10 5580; 1 University of New Mexico
Albuquerque, NM 87131-0001, USA

E-mail address:
wrayburn@salud.unm.edu

Obstet Gynecol Clin N Am 40 (2013) ix
http://dx.doi.org/10.1016/j.ogc.2013.01.001
0889-8545/13/$ – see front matter © 2013 Published by Elsevier Inc.

Preface

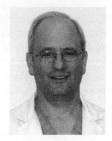

James M. Alexander, MD
Editor

Obstetric outcomes have improved dramatically in the last century. Maternal mortality, as high as 1% in 1930, is now reported to be between 7 and 15 per 100,000, an exponential decrease from before. Complications such as hypertensive stroke related to preeclampsia and renal failure due to obstetric hemorrhage are almost unheard of in modern practice. Today practitioners may not witness a maternal death their entire career. As a result of this improvement in outcome, elective interventions, including labor inductions and cesarean delivery on demand, have become commonplace and now third-party payors are limiting reimbursement when these interventions are too early and unindicated. Despite the safety of modern practice, obstetrics is still risky business and clinical scenarios develop that place the mother and fetus at risk. These obstetric emergencies develop suddenly and without immediate recognition; serious morbidity and even death can occur. This edition of the *Obstetrics and Gynecology Clinics* focuses on these obstetric emergencies and provides important information to the practicing obstetrician so that they can be recognized in a timely manner and appropriate therapy and treatment can be administered. Articles have been contributed that cover virtually all of the significant clinical obstetric emergencies encountered in practice today.

Sharon Phelan and Brad Holbrook have given us an update on how to manage cord prolapse, an unexpected, largely unpredictable event that can be disastrous. Alison Wortman and I have contributed an article on obstetric hemorrhage. Historically, hemorrhage has been one of the largest contributors to maternal death, and excessive blood loss at delivery is still a relatively common occurrence. Modern obstetric practice including improved blood banking techniques have greatly improved outcomes. We also contribute a related article on placenta accreta. Abnormal placentation is becoming more commonplace as the rate of cesarean delivery has increased and the slight increase in maternal mortality seen in recent years may be due to more of theses cases. Another diagnosis receiving increased attention in modern practice is embolic events. As mortality from the "big" three (hypertension, hemorrhage, and infection) has decreased, embolic events have become a more prominent cause of mortality. Drs Moore and Brennan have given us an important update on this subject including the latest information on both diagnosis and treatment. Drs Tyner and

Obstet Gynecol Clin N Am 40 (2013) xi–xii
http://dx.doi.org/10.1016/j.ogc.2013.01.002
0889-8545/13/$ – see front matter © 2013 Published by Elsevier Inc.

Rayburn have reminded us that emergent cesarean delivery, while lifesaving, is in and of itself associated with risk, and provided us with special precautions to minimize both morbidity and mortality.

Trauma is common and the leading cause of nonobstetric death. Drs Mozurkewich and Brown provide an important review on this subject. As pointed out by Dr Grobman in his article, shoulder dystocia is an uncommon and unpredictable event. His article provides important information on identification of the complication, maneuvers used to resolve it, and the use of simulation to minimize adverse outcome. Drs Roberts and Morgan have updated us on maternal sepsis. Although the more severe cases are often comanaged with other services in the ICU, the obstetricians' involvement is critical in the ultimate outcome. Dr Wilson and I have written an article on hypertensive crisis, a potentially life-threatening emergency that can lead to stroke, seizure, and other organ decompensation and failure. We also contribute an article about seizures and intracranial hemorrhage. Drs Sullivan and Goodier cover 2 endocrine emergencies, thyroid storm and diabetic ketoacidosis. Thyroid disease and diabetes are areas of current interest in our specialty and are the subject of active research. This article covers the more severe complications of these endocrine diseases.

I hope that this issue of *Obstetrics and Gynecology Clinics* will be of use to the clinician when faced with an obstetric emergency. In an era of improved maternal and fetal outcomes, where maternal mortality and fetal loss is uncommon, and where elective intervention is increasingly the norm, any of the emergencies discussed in this volume can catch one off guard. By recognizing the crisis and instituting immediate intervention and treatment, outcomes can be excellent for the mother and baby. This edition of the *Obstetrics and Gynecology Clinics* emphasizes this point over and over again.

I'd like to thank Elsevier and Dr William Rayburn for the opportunity to serve as guest editor for this issue and Stephanie Donley for all of her help.

James M. Alexander, MD
Department of Obstetrics and Gynecology
Division of Maternal Fetal Medicine
Parkland Hospital

E-mail address:
James.Alexander@UTSouthwestern.edu

Umbilical Cord Prolapse

Bradley D. Holbrook, MD*, Sharon T. Phelan, MD

KEYWORDS

- Umbilical cord prolapse • Obstetric emergency • Fetal hypoxia • Overt prolapse
- Occult prolapse

KEY POINTS

- Umbilical cord prolapse primarily happens in the setting of the rupture of membranes without a well-applied presenting fetal part, which includes situations with fetal malpresentation, iatrogenic elevation of fetal presentation, and anomalous fetus/cord.
- The occurrence of fetal bradycardia in the presence of ruptured membranes should prompt evaluation for possible cord prolapse.
- An expedited operative delivery is typically the treatment of choice, although the interval to delivery for a hospital-based prolapse is less critical than previously thought.
- When cesarean delivery cannot be done in a timely fashion, techniques that elevate the presenting part off the cord and keep the cord warm and moist may allow a safe transport to a location where an operative delivery can be done.
- In the setting of a previable or periviable pregnancy with a cord prolapse, conservative management may allow the pregnancy to continue to a more mature gestational age.

INTRODUCTION

Umbilical cord prolapse (UCP) is an obstetric emergency in which the umbilical cord comes through the cervical os in advance of or at the same time as the fetal presenting part. It can lead to poor fetal outcomes because it may cause the cord to be compressed between the fetus and the maternal bony pelvis or soft tissues, leading to fetal hypoxia.

There are 2 types of UCP. The first is overt prolapse, in which the cord prolapses in advance of the fetal presenting part and is palpable within the vagina or perhaps even visibly extruding from the vagina. In contrast, if the cord presents alongside the fetal presenting part but not below it, it is referred to as occult prolapse. The cord is not visible or palpable in occult prolapse.

The incidence of UCP ranges from 1.4 to 6.2 per 1000.[1] The rate has remained stable over the last century.[2] It is estimated that 77% of cases occur in singleton pregnancies; in twin pregnancies, 9% of cases occur in the first twin, and 14% in the second twin.[3]

Disclosures: The authors have nothing to disclose.
Department of Obstetrics and Gynecology, University of New Mexico School of Medicine, MSC 10 5580, 1 University of New Mexico, Albuquerque, NM 87131-0001, USA
* Corresponding author.
E-mail address: bholbrook@salud.unm.edu

Obstet Gynecol Clin N Am 40 (2013) 1–14
http://dx.doi.org/10.1016/j.ogc.2012.11.002
0889-8545/13/$ – see front matter © 2013 Elsevier Inc. All rights reserved.

obgyn.theclinics.com

In the past, UCP resulted in a high perinatal mortality, estimated at approximately 32% to 47% before the 1950s.[2] Since that time, the rate of perinatal mortality has decreased to 10% or less,[1,2,4,5] presumably because of the more widespread availability of cesarean delivery, as well as improved neonatal resuscitation and newborn care.

RISK FACTORS

Several risk factors have been identified that are associated with UCP. There are numerous studies that attempt to identify and rank these risk factors. However, because of the rare nature of UCP, even large-scale studies vary and disagree about the risk factors themselves, as well as the relative risk they incite. As such, this article does not attempt to assign a relative risk to each risk factor; it lists the recognized factors that may lead to an increased risk of UCP (**Box 1**). These factors can be separated into spontaneous and iatrogenic causes.

Spontaneous

Spontaneous umbilical cord prolapse can occur in otherwise uncomplicated pregnancies. These spontaneous causes share common characteristics: they are related to fetal or maternal conditions that prevent the fetus from being engaged in the pelvis or they occur because of abnormalities of the umbilical cord.

Of the spontaneous risk factors, fetal malpresentation is the most notable.[1] A fetus in an abnormal lie is less likely to be engaged in the maternal pelvis, thus allowing

---

Box 1
Risk factors for umbilical cord prolapse

Spontaneous

    Malpresentation

    Polyhydramnios

    Preterm delivery

    Preterm premature rupture of membranes

    Multiple gestation

    Fetal anomalies

    Grand multiparity

    Cord abnormalities

    Birth weight less than 2500 g

    Spontaneous rupture of membranes

Iatrogenic

    Amniotomy, especially with an unengaged fetal presenting part

    External cephalic version in a patient with ruptured membranes

    Attempted rotation of the fetal head (ie, occiput posterior to occiput anterior)

    Amnioinfusion

    Placement of an intrauterine pressure catheter or fetal scalp electrode

    Use of a cervical ripening balloon catheter

space for the cord to prolapse. Multiple gestation is also a known risk factor,[2] likely because of the increase in abnormal lie. Polyhydramnios[1,2] is an independent risk factor, although it is also associated with unstable lie and fetal anomalies, both of which are also spontaneous risk factors. Other fetal factors that increase the risk of UCP include preterm delivery,[2] as well as fetal growth restriction, or any reason for a birth weight less than 2500 g,[4] although there is some disagreement on this point[6] and some studies use less than 1500 g as the cutoff.[2] Spontaneous rupture of membranes is a risk factor, as is preterm premature rupture of membranes. Most cases of UCP occur shortly after rupture of membranes; one study found that 57% of cases occurred within 5 minutes of rupture, and 67% occur within 1 hour of rupture.[3] Only 5% of cases occur more than 24 hours after rupture.

Iatrogenic

Intrapartum interventions that are generally considered to be benign and routine for labor management have been identified as iatrogenic risk factors for UCP. Approximately 47% of cases of UCP can be attributed to iatrogenic factors.[3,7] Recognized iatrogenic factors tend to share one of two traits: they are either related to interventions that may cause the fetal presenting part to be elevated out of the pelvis or occur when rupturing the bag of waters.

These interventions include artificial rupture of membranes (especially if the fetal presenting part is not engaged), attempted rotation of the fetal head (ie, from occiput posterior to occiput anterior presentation), amnioinfusion, external cephalic version in a patient with ruptured membranes, placement of an intrauterine pressure catheter or fetal scalp electrode, or placement of a cervical ripening balloon catheter.

Despite a large percentage of cases of UCP being related to medical interventions, these iatrogenic causes are thought not to increase the associated perinatal morbidity and mortality because they are nearly always performed only on the labor and delivery unit, where the patient is likely undergoing continuous external fetal monitoring and where an urgent or emergent cesarean delivery can rapidly be performed. In addition, many of the iatrogenic risk factors are interventions that are used to treat spontaneous risk factors, and there is no evidence that these interventions increase the incidence of umbilical cord prolapse. Murphy and MacKenzie[3] note that the incidence of UCP is stable across populations, with no notable difference accountable to changes in obstetric practices.

DIAGNOSIS

Cord prolapse is diagnosed on examination, with an umbilical cord (usually a soft, pulsatile mass) being palpable within the vagina or visibly extruding from the introitus. It is often accompanied by a severe, sudden fetal heart rate deceleration with prolonged bradycardia or moderate to severe variable decelerations. However, these findings on fetal heart tracing are only present in 41% to 67% of cases.[3,4]

Overt cord prolapse is easier to diagnose than occult UCP, and it is likely that most cases of UCP reported in the literature are cases of overt prolapse. It is reasonable to assume that, for each case of overt prolapse, there may be multiple cases of occult cord prolapse that go undiagnosed; these would most likely result in a cesarean delivery for an unexplained fetal bradycardia. If the cord is not palpable, UCP cannot be definitively diagnosed.

However, even in cases of a palpable mass in the vagina, alternate diagnoses are possible and therefore must be considered. A palpable vaginal mass may be caused by an abnormal presentation such as a fetal limb, a face presentation, or severe caput succedaneum, and any of these could confuse a less experienced provider. In addition, in the case of a fetal demise, the mass may not be pulsatile.

In cases of severe, rapid fetal heart rate deceleration, a possible cord prolapse must be considered, although many other events may cause similar findings. Vaginal examination should be undertaken to evaluate for a visible or palpable cord. If either of these is present, the diagnosis is certain. Without a cord in the vagina, occult prolapse could still be present, but other causes of acute fetal bradycardia must be ruled out.

The most likely maternal factor to cause an acute, prolonged fetal heart rate deceleration would be maternal hypotension. Treatment of this condition is different than treatment of a prolapsed cord. Fluid resuscitation, pressor administration, and other interventions to treat the mother's cardiovascular status are also expected to resolve the fetal deceleration. This must be ruled out, particularly if the patient has just received spinal anesthesia.

Other fetal conditions could also cause sudden, prolonged decelerations and require urgent intervention. Vasa previa, placental abruption, and uterine rupture are other obstetric emergencies that may have a similar presentation to cord prolapse and also require immediate delivery.

PATHOPHYSIOLOGY

The cord prolapses out through the cervix because of the failure of the fetus to be engaged in the pelvis, thus allowing the cord to slip downward below the fetal presenting part after membranes are ruptured. The amniotic sac is at a higher pressure than the outside environment,[8] thus, when the membranes rupture, the fluid rushes out, aided by gravity in most cases. If the fetus is not engaged, a gap exists through which the cord may pass as it is swept downward with the rush of fluid.

Questions have been raised as to how much the cord is involved in the act of prolapsing. A cord that is thin or has little to no coiling and little Wharton jelly is at greater risk of being swept out through the cervix when membranes are ruptured. In addition to this, there have been two theories as to potential changes to the cord itself that may cause it to be more or less rigid, possibly predisposing it to prolapse. However, the two theories that attempt to explain this are in direct opposition to one another[9,10] and neither can be definitively supported; thus this aspect remains unclear.

The pathophysiology of the accompanying fetal heart rate deceleration is explained by normal physiologic function. The cord prolapses through the pelvic outlet in advance of the fetal presenting part. The forces of labor then cause the cord to be compressed between the fetus and the maternal bony pelvis, uterus, or cervix, which leads to compression of the umbilical arteries. In addition, vasospasm of the umbilical vessels may occur, probably because of the lower temperature of the vagina, and would exert a physiologic effect similar to external compression of the vessels.

Because an estimated 50% of the fetal circulation passes through the umbilical arteries,[11] compression of these arteries makes a large difference in the fetal cardiovascular status. Afterload is rapidly increased and the fetal heart must pump harder to overcome this increased vascular pressure. To increase pulse pressure, the heart rate must decline. This chain of events then leads to the classic findings on the fetal heart tracing: a sudden, severe reduction in the fetal heart rate.

Of course, the reduction in the fetal heart rate is not problematic in itself. The adverse fetal outcomes are a result of the fetal hypoxia that occurs because of impaired blood flow to and from the placenta; the shape of the abnormalities on fetal heart rate tracing are merely an indicator of the impaired flow, which, left untreated, may lead to poor outcomes.

PREVENTION

Because approximately half of all cases of cord prolapse are iatrogenic, it could be inferred that at least some cases are preventable. Although knowledge of risk factors has not been shown to reduce the risk of cord prolapse,[3] it is reasonable to exercise caution in certain situations that could lead to a cord prolapse. Even when the prolapse is not preventable, fetal morbidity and mortality can often be prevented.

Given the high risk of cord prolapse in malpresentation, a study was performed to evaluate cord presentation in breech deliveries. Although the current recommendation is that cesarean section is the preferred mode of delivery in cases of breech presentation,[12] this study was performed when breech vaginal delivery was more common. Study subjects who had fetuses in breech presentation at term were separated into two groups. One group received a transvaginal ultrasound to evaluate the location of the cord. No ultrasound was performed on the control group. More than 60% in both groups delivered vaginally without cord prolapse. Eight patients in the ultrasound group had a funic presentation and underwent cesarean delivery. There were no cases of cord prolapse in the ultrasound group. The group that did not receive an ultrasound had 10 cases of cord prolapse, 1 of which resulted in neonatal demise.[13]

At the same time, another study questioned whether antenatal ultrasound is useful. They reviewed 16 cases in which the cord was the presenting part on prenatal ultrasound. Repeating the ultrasound at a later date showed resolution in approximately 50% of cases. In addition, of the original 16 cases, only 2 experienced a cord prolapse.[14] Although it seems that a funic presentation as discovered on antepartum ultrasound does lead to an increased risk of cord prolapse, it is not clear that this justifies an intervention because it has a low predictive value for the benefit of prelabor intervention.

The act of rupturing the membranes, whether spontaneous or artificial, is a risk factor for cord prolapse. Thus, care must be used when undertaking such a procedure. If the fetal head is well applied on sterile vaginal examination, it is presumed that amniotomy may be performed safely. If not, amniotomy should be delayed. In cases in which it is thought that amniotomy must be performed despite an unengaged fetus, a controlled rupture should be performed, which should allow a slow release of fluid rather than the typical large, sudden decompression. Instead of using the routine hook, a hypodermic needle can be used. A pudendal block trumpet can be used to properly position the needle without risk of injuring maternal tissues. Once the trumpet is properly placed, the needle may be inserted and left in place while the amniotic fluid slowly drains through this controlled rupture in the bag of waters. The trumpet also holds the needle at a standard depth, thus decreasing the risk of the needle penetrating the sac too deeply and endangering the fetal head.

An unengaged fetal head is also a risk factor for cord prolapse. As such, vaginal manipulation of the fetal head must be performed with caution to avoid elevating the fetal head and thereby allowing space into which the cord may prolapse. Thus, with sterile vaginal examinations, as well as placement of a fetal scalp electrode or intrauterine pressure catheter, care must be taken not to elevate the fetal head more than is necessary to perform the procedure. Cervical ripening balloon catheters, by their nature, elevate the fetal head out of the pelvis and thus allow for the possibility of a cord prolapse. When placing a balloon catheter, there is little that can be done to avoid the possibility of a cord prolapse, but the clinician should understand that this intervention likely increases the risk that a prolapse may occur. For this reason, many physicians recommend against placing a cervical ripening balloon catheter if the patient's membranes are already ruptured, although there is some disagreement in the literature regarding this.[15] Overall, care should be used with any of the procedures mentioned earlier. Furthermore, they should only be performed when other methods are not sufficient, and not simply as part of routine labor monitoring.

Another important consideration is preventing fetal morbidity or mortality from UCP in cases in which the prolapse may not be preventable. Patients with high risk of umbilical cord prolapse based on the risk factors described earlier, as well as patients with funic presentations seen on ultrasound, should be counseled by their providers regarding the risk of UCP. They should be given strict precautions to present immediately for evaluation with rupture of membranes or decreased fetal movement. Such counseling may lead to more rapid presentation in cases of UCP and thus may improve outcomes.

One high-risk group for development of UCP is patients with preterm premature rupture of membranes (PPROM). A study of inpatient versus outpatient management of PPROM found that inpatient management decreases risk of perinatal morbidity and mortality from UCP, among other issues that may arise.[16] Thus, although inpatient management of PPROM does little to prevent the act of cord prolapse, the presence of the patient in the hospital allows urgent intervention to prevent problems when this emergency does occur.

Intrapartum continuous external fetal heart rate monitoring should similarly be used in patients with risk factors for UCP. Some form of heart rate monitoring is used in approximately 85% of deliveries.[17] In many facilities, continuous monitoring is the norm, although data support intermittent auscultation, and its use is accepted by the American College of Obstetricians and Gynecologists.[17] However, in cases with the known risk factors for cord prolapse listed earlier, intermittent auscultation is contraindicated because it may delay recognition and intervention if a cord prolapse does occur. Thus, we recommend the use of continuous electronic fetal monitoring should risk factors exist.

MANAGEMENT
Immediate Delivery

Cord prolapse can quickly lead to fetal compromise, with resultant long-term disability or death.[2,4,18] As such, cases of cord prolapse should be delivered as quickly as possible. In general, this requires cesarean delivery. However, in rare cases in which the first stage of labor is already complete and it is thought that vaginal delivery would likely be more rapidly achieved than cesarean delivery, spontaneous or operative vaginal delivery may be performed. The decision for operative versus spontaneous delivery should depend on the fetal heart tracing.

The primary management until delivery can be performed is funic decompression (ie, relieving the pressure on the umbilical cord from the fetal presenting part). There are different procedures described to achieve this same goal. Even in cases in which immediate delivery is possible, funic decompression should be performed for as long as possible until delivery occurs.

Pressure on the cord can be relieved by the physician placing two fingers, or the entire hand if possible, into the patient's vagina and gently elevating the fetal presenting part. While doing this, extreme care is taken to avoid putting further pressure on the cord. Even light palpation of the cord should be avoided because it can cause vasospasm and thus lead to a worse outcome.[2]

The patient should also be positioned to allow gravity to aid in decompressing the cord. Thus, the patient should be placed in either steep Trendelenburg or knee-chest position until she is able to deliver.[19]

In addition to gravity, the patient's anatomy may be manipulated to decrease pressure on the cord. Placing a Foley catheter and instilling saline into the bladder can successfully elevate the fetal presenting part off the cord. This was first suggested by Vago[20] in 1970. He presented a brief case series describing his success in using bladder instillation in cases in which vaginal delivery was not imminent. He described the then-current maneuvers, which included positional changes as well as manual elevation of the fetus with the physician's hand in the vagina. He noted that vaginal elevation is "effective, but is unpleasant for the mother and wearying for the doctor." His procedure was to instill 500 to 750 mL of normal saline into the bladder using a Foley catheter, which is then clamped to maintain distention of the bladder. To determine the necessary quantity of saline, he proposed that it be instilled until the distended bladder is visible as a swelling above the pubis, noting that 500 mL are usually sufficient. The distended bladder then provides upward pressure on the fetal presenting part, thus relieving the life-threatening compression. He also noted the additional benefit that, in his experience, filling the bladder also leads to calming of uterine contractions.

Over time, Vago's method has proved to be effective.[20,21] Thus, this method is preferred in cases of expected prolonged interval to delivery, because it is more tolerable, both to the patient and the clinician, than continuous elevation of the fetal presenting part with the clinician's hand in the patient's vagina.

In one case series, a prolonged interval to cesarean delivery was managed with Vago's method only. There were no cases of neonatal death.[21] At the same time, if cesarean delivery can be performed promptly, Vago's method has been shown to provide no advantage compared with manual elevation of the fetal head, and the combination of the two methods leads to no improvement compared with manual elevation alone.[22] However, bladder filling can potentially allow spinal anesthesia and a calmer, controlled cesarean delivery instead of an emergent cesarean delivery under general anesthesia. In cases in which the anticipated diagnosis-to-delivery interval (DDI) is prolonged, filling the bladder should be used.

Another management modality that is currently used only rarely is replacement of the umbilical cord into the uterus, above the fetal presenting part. This procedure is known as funic reduction. Its use was common before the widespread availability of cesarean delivery. However, outcomes were generally poor. Barrett[23] notes that these poor outcomes were also in an era before fetal monitoring became widely available, and that its use has not been reevaluated since continuous fetal heart monitoring has been available.

Barrett[23] reports his personal experience of 8 cases of UCP over a 10-year period (during which he delivered 2188 infants). Cases of UCP were managed with funic reduction. The technique is to gently elevate the fetal head using a hand in the vagina, then digitally lift the cord above the fetal head at its widest point, with the goal of replacing the cord in the nuchal region. He recommends the use of an assistant who can provide suprapubic pressure; the goal of this is, first, to assist in elevating he fetal head off the umbilical cord, and, second, to help hold the fetus in a cephalic presentation, thereby decreasing the chance of version to a malpresentation. Continuous fetal monitoring should be used during and after the procedure, and, while the procedure is being performed, preparations should be underway to perform a cesarean delivery in case it is unsuccessful.

Of his 8 patients with UCP, all neonates were live born and had normal Apgar scores at 5 minutes. One patient did require a cesarean delivery because the cervix was not adequately dilated for him to perform the reduction. In addition, 2 cases did not undergo funic reduction because vaginal delivery was deemed to be imminent. In the 5 cases in which he attempted funic reduction, he was able to successfully replace the cord, and interval to delivery ranged from 14 to 512 minutes. Each of these successful cases had had a prior successful vaginal delivery, and only a short segment of cord had prolapsed. The procedure would likely be more difficult and the chances of success would likely diminish if it were performed in a primipara or if the prolapsed cord were long. Overall, Barrett[23] notes a cesarean section rate of only 12.5%, lower than that of other studies. However, his short-term neonatal outcomes were as good as those studies of emergent cesarean delivery. Given his good outcomes in this small case series, he recommends attempted funic reduction in cases of cord prolapse with a short segment of cord (<25 cm), with cervical dilation greater than or equal to 4 cm, ability to elevate the fetal vertex above −1 station. It should be completed within 2 minutes. The fetal heart rate should return to normal once it is complete. Continuous fetal monitoring is necessary. While performing the funic reduction, preparations should be made for cesarean delivery.

Administration of a tocolytic agent has also been proposed as an adjunct to elevation of the fetal presenting part. Katz and colleagues[19] described backfilling the bladder and then administering an intravenous infusion of ritodrine (Yutopar; a β-mimetic that is no longer available in the United States), theorizing that decreasing uterine tone and contractions would further relieve pressure on the prolapsed cord. In addition, they thought that a tocolytic is also likely to increase placental perfusion and thus lead to improved fetal outcomes. Like many of the studies discussed earlier, Katz and colleagues[19] reported excellent fetal outcomes. In their 12 cases, they had no fetal or neonatal deaths and Apgar scores at 5 minutes ranged from 7 to 10. One criticism of the use of a tocolytic is that it may lead to uterine atony after delivery is accomplished. Katz and colleagues[19] reported mild hypotonicity of the uterus after delivery in 2 cases, but noted that both of these resolved with administration of oxytocin.

Overall, it seems that tocolysis may be a useful adjunct, but is not a primary treatment. It does not seem to be necessary in cases in which immediate delivery can be accomplished; this is noted by Katz and colleagues.[19] In cases of prolonged interval to delivery, tocolysis may or may not be necessary. We recommend first initiating the first-line therapies noted earlier, considering administration of a tocolytic agent only if fetal distress persists with delivery not being imminent.

In summary, the primary management of UCP is immediate delivery. Once UCP has been diagnosed, the most rapid method of delivery should be performed. If vaginal delivery is imminent, spontaneous or operative vaginal delivery can be performed. Otherwise, preparations should be made for urgent cesarean delivery. In the interval to delivery, the patient should be placed in Trendelenburg or knee-chest position and the fetal presenting part elevated to alleviate cord compression, either by placing a hand in the vagina to elevate the fetal presenting part, or by filling the bladder.

Prolonged Interval to Delivery

There are situations in which immediate delivery is not possible or is not desirable. The most obvious example is cord prolapse in a rural setting or a birthing center, where resources to perform cesarean deliveries do not exist. In cases in which immediate delivery is not an option, extreme care must be taken to minimize fetal risk while transporting mother and child to a location where delivery can be performed.

In cases of anticipated prolonged interval to delivery, it is important to minimize cord compression. This can be done through the methods described earlier. Thus, the patient should be placed in Trendelenburg or knee-chest position and the fetal presenting part elevated. For the comfort of both the patient and provider, bladder filling seems to be a better option to elevate the fetal presenting part if the interval to delivery is expected to be long.[20] Fetal heart monitoring should be performed. If bradycardia persists, a tocolytic can be administered, and, if it does not resolve after tocolysis, an attempt at funic reduction is reasonable.[23]

Another important consideration in cases of prolonged interval to delivery is keeping the cord moist. If the cord is extruded from the vagina, it may dry out and thus impair blood flow. It has also been postulated that the lower temperature in the vagina or outside the introitus may lead to vasospasm, thus also impairing blood flow. If the cord is extruded from the vagina, it may be replaced into the vagina and a moist tampon or Kerlix gently inserted to hold it in place.[19]

Expectant Management

Although urgent delivery is nearly always the treatment of choice for UCP, there are contraindications to immediate delivery (**Box 2**). If the fetus has lethal anomalies, there is nothing to be gained by urgent delivery. Similarly, if fetal heart tones are absent, a demise has already occurred, and submitting the mother to the risks of a cesarean delivery will yield no additional benefit. In addition, cases of UCP at a previable gestational age should not be delivered. The age of viability varies greatly based on institutional policies and neonatal intensive care unit (NICU) facilities.

Leong and colleagues[24] presented a single case report of prolonged expectant management of cord prolapse. The patient presented to the hospital at 23 weeks and 1 day's gestation and had hourglassing membranes that ruptured on the same day. On examination, a cord was visible within the vagina. Because of the extreme prematurity, expectant management was undertaken. The patient received antibiotics and corticosteroids and was placed on bed rest, with the goal of prolonging pregnancy until 26 weeks' gestation. The umbilical cord prolapsed out of the vagina on several occasions, usually after a bowel movement, and was digitally replaced each time. Once the patient reached 26 weeks and 1 day's gestation, she was delivered via classical cesarean section. Apgar scores were 6 at 5 minutes and 7 at 10 minutes. The infant required long-term oxygen because of lung disease from prematurity, but no other long-term complications were reported.

There is a similar case of UCP caused by extreme prematurity that was managed expectantly for 2 weeks with similarly good neonatal outcome.[2] Thus, in rare cases such as these, prolonged expectant management may be indicated.

OUTCOMES

Overall, neonatal outcomes in cases of cord prolapse are good. If the prolapse occurs while in the hospital and near medical care, the outcomes are better, whereas if it occurs at a remote location, there is more morbidity and mortality. One study showed an 18-fold increase in perinatal mortality in cases of cord prolapse occurring outside the hospital, even compared with an unmonitored fetus whose cord prolapsed while in the hospital.[4] Overall, nearly all neonates delivered within 30 minutes do well.[3] However, a short DDI has been shown to be less important if the prolapse occurs while

---

Box 2
Contraindications to immediate delivery in cases of umbilical cord prolapse

Lethal fetal anomalies

Previable gestation

Fetal demise

the patient is already in the hospital[3]; this is presumably a result of immediate intervention to relieve cord compression.

Murphy and MacKenzie[3] performed a study to evaluate long-term outcomes following cases of UCP, 3 years from the time of delivery. They found that infants born vaginally tended to have shorter DDIs and better Apgar scores than their counterparts born via cesarean section, although blood gas values were virtually the same. This may be confounded by those infants who underwent a vaginal delivery likely being near delivery to begin with and having fetal heart tracings that were reassuring enough that the provider was comfortable proceeding with a vaginal delivery. The investigators also noted that the interval to delivery had little effect on Apgar scores if they delivered within 30 minutes. However, as the interval passed 30 minutes, scores began to decrease.

In this study, only 1 infant did not survive as a direct result of the cord prolapse; the other deaths were caused by prematurity, lethal anomalies, and placental abruption. Of the 120 surviving newborns, only 1 had cerebral palsy, and he was extremely premature. From these findings, they inferred that it is unlikely that acute hypoxia for 30 to 60 minutes is directly responsible for long-term neurologic damage.[3]

At the same time, more recent studies have cast doubt on whether the DDI is the most important predictor of neonatal outcome. In a case series of 44 patients with cord prolapse, the mean time to delivery was 18 minutes. Thirteen of those deliveries (29%) required transfer of the infant to the NICU and had Apgar scores of less than 7 at 5 minutes. Ten of the 13 (76%) had delivered within 18 minutes. However, most of those patients were rushed to the operating room with no additional procedures performed; only 12 (27%) underwent some maneuver to alleviate pressure on the cord.[25] Most of these neonates were born prematurely, which could also lead to transfer to the NICU for reasons unrelated to UCP.

This study implies that intervention to elevate the fetal presenting part off the cord may be more important than the interval to delivery. In addition, other factors that are more difficult to quantify, such as the severity of cord compression and presence of any underlying fetal compromise, may also have a bearing on the outcome.

The DDI seems to be less important in cases of UCP associated with PPROM at less than 34 weeks' gestation, with the patient not in active labor, likely because of the lack of uterine contractions. However, the physical properties of the umbilical cord change with advancing gestation, with a decreased propensity to coil, as well as a decrease in

---

Box 3
Key components of team simulation training for umbilical cord prolapse

Include all medical staff involved in labor and delivery

Training should be required annually, with training dates spread throughout the year

Each team member's role and responsibility should be clearly outlined

Simulated emergencies should be rehearsed, using patient-actors as well as plastic models

Objectives of the course should be to teach participants to:

• Recognize risk factors for umbilical cord prolapse

• Call for assistance

• Perform appropriate maneuvers to alleviate compression of the cord

• Communicate effectively with the patient and her family

• Document appropriately

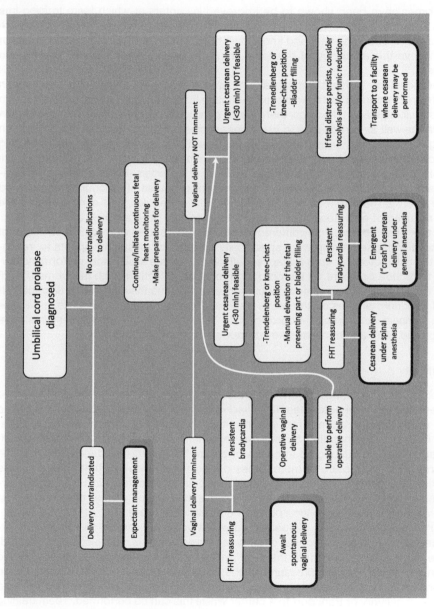

Fig. 1. Algorithm for the management of umbilical cord prolapse. FHT, fetal heart tracing.

hyaluronan. It is possible that, because of these changes, the preterm cord may be protected from compressive forces compared with a term cord.[26]

SIMULATION TRAINING

Outcomes have been shown to be improved in centers at which team training has been undertaken. Simulations or drills have been used to ensure that all parties are prepared for such an event and know their roles. Such team training has been shown to improve the efficiency of the team, thus decreasing the time from prolapse to delivery.[27]

Another study showed that similar simulation training was able to reduce the mean DDI from 25 minutes to 14.5 minutes. Although there were too few cases to draw firm statistically significant findings, there was a trend toward increased use of spinal anesthesia, as well as a reduction in low Apgar scores and NICU admissions.[28] Although a larger-scale study needs to be performed to verify these findings, these team training exercises may lead to improved neonatal outcomes.

This study included a multidisciplinary team of midwives, obstetricians, and anesthetists, all of whom underwent a 1-day training course. This course was offered once every 2 months to accommodate different schedules, and annual attendance was required of each team member; compliance was between 95% and 100%.

At the 1-day course, many different obstetric emergencies were simulated. Goals of the cord prolapse training were specifically defined, to "teach participants to: recognise the risk factors for cord prolapse; call for appropriate assistance; perform maneuvers to reduce pressure on the cord; communicate effectively with the woman; [and] take detailed contemporaneous documentation." During the day, the participants fulfilled their normal roles on the team. Patient-actors were used in the drills, as well as fetal, perineal, and umbilical cord models. After each drill, feedback sessions were performed. **Box 3** summarizes key components of simulation training.

SUMMARY

Umbilical cord prolapse is an obstetric emergency that, untreated, can lead to extremely poor fetal outcomes. It is diagnosed by a palpable cord within the vagina or a visible cord extruded from the introitus in the setting of ruptured membranes, and is often accompanied by severe, rapid fetal heart rate decelerations. Occult prolapse may be suspected in cases of severe fetal heart rate decelerations in the setting of recent rupture of membranes or obstetric maneuvers that might increase the risk of prolapse. Risk factors include malpresentation, low birth weight, polyhydramnios, prematurity, and iatrogenic causes at the time of any intervention that may cause the fetal presenting part to be displaced upward.

When cord prolapse is suspected, a sterile vaginal examination should be performed to confirm the diagnosis; other competing diagnoses must also be considered. If the diagnosis is confirmed, the fetal presenting part should be elevated with the vaginal hand to alleviate pressure on the cord. Delivery should take place as soon as possible; if vaginal delivery is not imminent, preparations must be made for rapid cesarean delivery or transport to a center where this can be performed. Team training exercises have been shown to decrease the diagnosis-to-delivery interval and seem to lead to improved neonatal outcomes. Although an urgent cesarean delivery is indicated, an emergent procedure likely subjects the mother to significant risk of morbidity without significant improvement in fetal outcome if the fetal presenting part has been appropriately displaced from off the cord.

While awaiting delivery, the patient should be placed in steep Trendelenburg position or knee-chest position. If the interval to delivery is likely to be prolonged, filling the bladder with 500 to 700 mL of saline has been shown to be effective in reducing cord compressions as well. If the fetal heart tracing does not recover, administration of a tocolytic agent may be considered. Funic reduction is a controversial procedure that may have benefit but has not been adequately studied. Management is summarized in **Fig. 1**.

Although an untreated case of umbilical cord prolapse can lead to severe fetal morbidity and mortality, prompt and appropriate management leads to good overall outcomes.

REFERENCES

1. Kahana B, Sheiner E, Levy A, et al. Umbilical cord prolapse and perinatal outcomes. Int J Gynaecol Obstet 2004;84(2):127–32.
2. Lin MG. Umbilical cord prolapse. Obstet Gynecol Surv 2006;61(4):269–77.
3. Murphy DJ, MacKenzie IZ. The mortality and morbidity associated with umbilical cord prolapse. Br J Obstet Gynaecol 1995;102(10):826–30.
4. Koonings PP, Paul RH, Campbell K. Umbilical cord prolapse: a contemporary look. J Reprod Med 1990;35(7):690–2.
5. Boyle JJ, Katz VL. Umbilical cord prolapse in current obstetric practice. J Reprod Med 2005;50(5):303–6.
6. Uygur D, Kis S, Tuncer R, et al. Risk factors and infant outcomes associated with umbilical cord prolapse. Int J Gynaecol Obstet 2002;78(2):127–30.
7. Usta IM, Mercer BM, Sibai BM. Current obstetrical practice and umbilical cord prolapse. Am J Perinatol 1999;16(9):479–84.
8. Fisk NM, Tannirandorn Y, Nicolini U, et al. Amniotic pressure in disorders of amniotic fluid volume. Obstet Gynecol 1990;76(2):210–4.
9. Clark DO, Copeland W, Ullery JC. Prolapse of the umbilical cord. A study of 117 cases. Am J Obstet Gynecol 1968;101(1):84–90.
10. McDaniels HR, Umezaki H, Harer WB, et al. Is umbilical cord prolapse secondary to fetal acidemia? Prenat Neonatal Med 2001;6(2):129–32.
11. Fineman JR, Clyman R. Fetal cardiovascular physiology. In: Creasy RK, Resnick R, Iams JD, editors. Creasy and Resnick's maternal-fetal medicine: principles and practice. 6th edition. Philadelphia: Saunders Elsevier; 2009. p. 161–2.
12. ACOG Committee on Obstetric Practice. ACOG committee opinion no. 340. Mode of term singleton breech delivery. Obstet Gynecol 2006;108(1):235–7.
13. Kinugasa M. Antepartum detection of cord presentation by transvaginal ultrasound for term breech presentation: potential prediction and prevention of cord prolapse. J Obstet Gynaecol Res 2007;33(5):612–8.
14. Ezra Y, Strasberg SR, Farine D. Does cord presentation on ultrasound predict cord prolapse? Gynecol Obstet Invest 2003;56(1):6–9.
15. Wolff K, Swahn ML, Westgren M. Balloon catheter for induction of labor in nulliparous women with prelabor rupture of the membranes at term. A preliminary report. Gynecol Obstet Invest 1998;46(1):1–4.
16. Ellestad SC, Swamy GK, Sinclair T, et al. Preterm premature rupture of membrane management—inpatient versus outpatient: a retrospective review. Am J Perinatol 2008;25(1):69–73.
17. American College of Obstetricians and Gynecologists. ACOG practice bulletin no. 106: intrapartum fetal heart rate monitoring: nomenclature, interpretation, and general management principles. Obstet Gynecol 2009;114(1):192–202.

18. Critchlow CW, Leet TL, Benedetti TJ, et al. Risk factors and infant outcomes associated with umbilical cord prolapse: a population-based case-control study among births in Washington State. Am J Obstet Gynecol 1994;170(2):613–8.
19. Katz Z, Lancet M, Borenstein R. Management of labor with umbilical cord prolapse. Am J Obstet Gynecol 1982;142(2):239–41.
20. Vago T. Prolapse of the umbilical cord. Am J Obstet Gynecol 1970;107:967.
21. Caspi E, Lotan Y, Schrever PL. Prolapse of the cord: reduction of perinatal mortality by bladder instillation and cesarean section. Isr J Med Sci 1983;19(6):541–5.
22. Bord I, Gemer O, Anteby EY, et al. The value of bladder filling in addition to manual elevation of presenting fetal part in cases of cord prolapse. Arch Gynecol Obstet 2011;283(5):989–91.
23. Barrett JM. Funic reduction for the management of umbilical cord prolapse. Am J Obstet Gynecol 1991;165(3):654–7.
24. Leong A, Rao J, Opie G, et al. Fetal survival after conservative management of cord prolapse for three weeks. BJOG 2004;111(12):1476–7.
25. Khan RS, Naru T, Nizami F. Umbilical cord prolapse—a review of diagnosis to delivery interval on perinatal and maternal outcome. J Pak Med Assoc 2007;57(10):487–91.
26. Nizard J, Cromi A, Molendijk H, et al. Neonatal outcome following prolonged umbilical cord prolapse in preterm premature rupture of membranes. BJOG 2005;112(6):833–6.
27. Tan WC, Tan LK, Tan HK, et al. Audit of "crash" emergency caesarean sections due to cord prolapse in terms of response time and perinatal outcomes. Ann Acad Med Singap 2003;32(5):638–41.
28. Siassakos D, Hasafa Z, Sibanda T, et al. Retrospective cohort study of diagnosis-delivery interval with umbilical cord prolapse: the effect of team training. BJOG 2009;116(8):1089–96.

Intrapartum Hemorrhage

James M. Alexander, MD*, Alison C. Wortman, MD

KEYWORDS

- Hemorrhage • Uterine atony • Abruption • Resuscitation • Transfusion

KEY POINTS

- Learning to recognize the signs and symptoms of shock and familiarization with techniques for treatment and resuscitation are critical to successful outcome.
- Obstetric hemorrhage can be classified as antepartum, intrapartum, and postpartum.
- The first key to management of intrapartum hemorrhage is to recognize its occurrence in a timely fashion.
- Management may include medical or surgical approaches or a combination of both.

Hemorrhage is commonly encountered in obstetric practice and is at times deadly. Historically, hemorrhage, along with hypertension and infection, have been the largest contributors to maternal mortality, which as recently as 1930 was 1% in the United States and Britain.[1,2] Although the overall risk of death in childbirth is now greatly diminished, hemorrhage remains a major causative factor. Clark and colleagues[3] reported on the causes of maternal death among 1.5 million deliveries from 2000 to 2006 and 12% were related to obstetric hemorrhage. Hemorrhage was the direct cause of death in 17% of the more than 4000 pregnancy-related deaths in the United States as reported by the Pregnancy Mortality Surveillance System of the Centers for Disease Control and Prevention.[4,5] In the world, hemorrhage has been reported as the single most common cause of death and accounts for more than half of all deaths worldwide.[6,7]

Although maternal mortality is low in the United States, there many have been a recent increase. The Joint Commission on Accreditation of Healthcare Organizations issued a sentinel event alert in 2010 in response to an increase in maternal mortality from 6 per 100,000 to 13 to 15 per 100,000.[8] Although the rates are still quite low by historical standards, any increase is concerning when one recognizes the great improvements seen over the past 80 or so years.[1] The recent increase in maternal mortality is likely multifactorial and related to increased maternal age at delivery and the associated comorbidities, improved management of chronic disease, and

Department of Obstetrics and Gynecology, University of Texas Southwestern Medical Center, 5323 Harry Hines Boulevard, Dallas, TX 75390-9032, USA
* Corresponding author.
E-mail address: James.Alexander@UTSouthwestern.edu

Obstet Gynecol Clin N Am 40 (2013) 15–26
http://dx.doi.org/10.1016/j.ogc.2012.12.003
0889-8545/13/$ – see front matter © 2013 Elsevier Inc. All rights reserved.

increased elective interventions that result in an increased cesarean delivery rate. The latter greatly increases the risk of placenta accreta and may explain in part increased deaths due to obstetric hemorrhage.[9] This is addressed in detail in the article by Wortman elsewhere in this issue.

Obstetric hemorrhage can be classified as antepartum, intrapartum, and postpartum. Antepartum hemorrhage is seen in placenta previa and sometimes abruption. Intrapartum hemorrhage is the focus of this article and has several causes and predisposing factors, as shown in **Box 1**. Many of these causes, such as uterine atony, are also associated with postpartum hemorrhage, which is usually immediate, although sometimes can be delayed. Increased risk of intrapartum hemorrhage from placenta accreta has been recently seen and is related to the unprecedented rise in cesarean deliveries. Although placenta accreta can be seen in an unscarred uterus, a cesarean delivery greatly increases the risk in subsequent pregnancies.[8,9]

INTRAPARTUM HEMORRHAGE

The consequences of intrapartum hemorrhage are related to the degree of blood loss and the timeliness of resuscitative measures. The uterus at full gestation receives 600 mL of blood per minute, placing the woman at risk for massive amounts of blood loss in a short amount of time, a true obstetric emergency.[10] The physiologic response to hemorrhage in the pregnant woman is no different from other patients experiencing acute blood loss. Initially, cardiac output, stroke volume, and mean arterial blood pressure decrease, tissue oxygen extraction increases, and pulmonary capillary wedge pressure falls. Redistribution of blood flow occurs through selective, arteriolar-mediated vasoconstriction and results in diminished perfusion to the kidneys, skin, and uterus while maintaining flow to the heart and brain. Cardiac output is maintained,

---

Box 1
Some causes and predisposing factors of obstetric hemorrhage

Abnormal placentation

- Previa
- Abruption
- Accreta

Injury during labor and delivery

- Vaginal or cervical laceration
- Uterine rupture
- Uterine laceration during cesarean delivery

Uterine atony

- Overdistended uterus
  - Macrosomia
  - Multiple gestation
  - Polyhydramnios
- Labor induction
- Prolonged labor
- Rapid labor

through increases in the heart rate and contractility. Systemic vascular resistance increases as well. Adequate resuscitative measures during this initial response will quickly reverse the developing shock and full recovery will typically be seen if the source of the hemorrhage is identified and controlled.

If the blood volume deficit exceeds 25 volume percent, cardiac output and blood pressure will begin to drop and there will be rapid clinical deterioration.[11–14] The initial benefits of redistribution of blood flow will be lost as cellular hypoxia and death begin to occur in the organs that blood flow is being shunted away from. The resultant tissue and organ damage lead to an inflammatory response and endothelial activation. This endothelial involvement leads to loss of the integrity of the vascular wall, increased cell membrane permeability, and capillary leak.

Pregnancy has a couple of advantages when compared with other clinical scenarios, both related to maternal age and pregnancy-related maternal adaptation, which includes volume expansion. The average maternal age at delivery is 24 years and occurs at a time in life when women are at their peak physiologic condition.[4] Women at this age are typically healthy and do not have significant comorbidities. Unlike other patient populations, women who are pregnant handle moderate amounts of hemorrhage well and usually recover unscathed. More importantly than this, the adaptation of blood volume to pregnancy confers a protective advantage against excessive blood loss that is unique. This volume expansion begins at the end of the first trimester and results in a 50% increase in the blood volume, which leads to an additional 1000 to 1500 mL of circulating blood volume at the time of delivery. Considering that the average blood loss at vaginal delivery is 500 mL and at cesarean delivery is 1000 mL, most women have ample reserve at term for routine blood loss and moderate amounts of hemorrhage.[15]

There are some conditions in which maternal volume expansion does not occur. Women with preeclampsia typically have decreased plasma volumes as compared with those who do not have preeclampsia.[16] The degree of contraction appears to be related to the severity of disease and has been reported to be a 50% decrease from normal in nulliparous women with eclampsia. There continues to be debate about whether this occurs after clinical onset of the disease and is really a volume constriction or if the changes occur before the onset of disease. Chronic renal disease has also been associated with abnormal volume expansion. The consequence of this is profound, as these women will not tolerate hemorrhage and even the normal blood loss seen at delivery may result in decompensation and hemorrhagic shock.

IDENTIFICATION OF EXCESSIVE BLOOD LOSS

The first key to management of intrapartum hemorrhage is to recognize its occurrence in a timely fashion. Bleeding often begins at the time of placental separation, and although it can be brisk and obvious, it is sometimes more subtle and can be steady and relentless. In the face of other bodily fluids associated with delivery, including ammonic and urine that are also present, the amount of blood loss is often underestimated. Pritchard and colleagues[17] reported that the estimated blood loss is commonly only half the actual loss. Although techniques such as calibrated drape markings can improve accuracy, underestimation is still common.[18,19] The steady bleeding seen initially appears moderate, but will persist until serious hypovolemia has occurred. Further complicating this is the failure of the pulse and blood pressure to change significantly until large amounts of blood have been lost. In fact, as peripheral vasoconstriction occurs and shunting of blood to the core organs begins, the woman may initially become hypertensive.[20] This may be particularly pronounced in preeclampsia where the blood pressure is already high. One of the most accurate measures of the degree of blood loss is urine output. The kidneys are particularly sensitive to acute blood loss and subsequent hypovolemia and will decrease urine production relatively quickly. Ultimately, experience may be the most significant factor in identifying hemorrhage quickly. Because of the subtleties involved in the initial diagnosis of excessive blood loss, it is often the appreciation that it is "more than normal" that prompts recognition of the blood loss and the emergency at hand.

Once identified, resuscitative measures should be quickly taken including obtaining intravenous access with 2 large-bore intravenous lines for rapid infusion of crystalloid and blood, placement of a Foley catheter to monitor urine output, an effort made to identify the cause (ie, uterine atony, genital laceration, or other diagnoses) and mobilization of surgical and anesthesia teams as needed.

CAUSES OF HEMORRHAGE

The cause of intrapartum hemorrhage can include placenta previa, accreta abruption, uterine atony that occurs immediately after delivery, uterine injury and laceration, vaginal or cervical laceration, and vaginal hematoma. Although labor can initiate the bleeding that occurs with a placenta previa, this more often occurs spontaneously and antepartum, so is not considered here. Accreta is also not commented on here, as it is covered in the article by Wortman elsewhere in this issue. Abruption is most often categorized as an antepartum event; however, because it is so often associated with labor, and the coagulopathy that ensues greatly complicates intrapartum management, it is covered in this article. Management of intrapartum hemorrhage is medical or surgical depending on the cause; medical management is covered with postpartum atony and surgical management is discussed after uterine, cervical, and vaginal injury and laceration.

Abruption

Abruption is the diagnosis given when the placenta separates from the uterus before the onset of labor. The bleeding that occurs is a result of this blood tracking between the membranes and uterus until it passes through the cervix. Often, a large amount of the blood lost is retained between the detached placenta and uterus, where it is concealed. Large amounts of blood can build up here and the extent of hemorrhage is usually not fully appreciated until delivery.[21] The morbidity of an abruption is not only related to the volume of blood loss, but is also related to the coagulopathy that develops.

In one-third of abruptions severe enough to kill the fetus, significant hypofibrinogenemia occurs (fibrinogen levels of less than 150 mg/dL). This is because of tissue thromboplastin released into the maternal venous bloodstream.[22,23] Abnormal activation of the extrinsic intravascular coagulation cascade and massive fibrinolysis then ensues. Fibrinogen-fibrin degradation products and d-dimers are seen and thrombocytopenia sometimes occurs. Delivery of the fetus stops the process and the abnormal coagulation status will correct itself relatively quickly, with appropriate resuscitation and transfusion of blood products. A vaginal delivery can be ideal as the uterus does not require an intact coagulation system for hemostasis; however, the fetus will not always tolerate labor in an abruption, and a cesarean will be required for fetal indication. When a cesarean delivery is required, significant bleeding will occur from the surgery if appropriate replacement of clotting factors does not occur. In abruption cases associated with a stillbirth, vaginal delivery is always preferred because of the coagulopathy so often present.[22,24]

Placental abruption occurs in 1 of every 200 deliveries. The National Center for Health Statistics reports an incidence of 1 in 160 in singleton gestations, and US birth certificate data from 2003 showed an incidence of 1 in 190 deliveries.[4,25] Parkland hospital has reported a decrease in abruptions severe enough to kill a fetus from 1 in 420 between 1956 and 1967 to 1 in 1600 in the years between 1996 and 2003.[21] Abruptions are most commonly associated with hypertension and abdominal trauma, but all of the following risk factors have been reported[26–31]:

- Maternal age older than 40
- African American or Caucasian race
- Premature rupture of the membranes
- Smoking
- Cocaine
- Leiomyomas
- Previous abruption
- Polyhydramnios

The management of abruption once identified is to effect delivery. If the fetus is alive, then a cesarean delivery will often be necessary, unless vaginal delivery is imminent or the abruption affects a small part of the placenta. Two very important caveats must be kept in mind:

- The blood loss may be much greater than is evident on vaginal/cervical examination
- A coagulopathy may be present even though clinical evidence may be lacking

With adequate resuscitative measures using crystalloid blood products, including red blood cells, plasma, and even platelets, the maternal outcome can be excellent even in cases in which the fetus is lost.

Although effecting delivery is necessary to resolve the abruption and save the fetus, delaying the delivery if the fetus is premature is sometimes beneficial.[32,33] Bond and associates[32] demonstrated a benefit to expectant management at less than 35 weeks with a reported 12-day delay in delivery from the time of diagnosis. No stillbirths were reported and most deliveries were by cesarean. This management should be approached with trepidation, and decompensation of the fetus may be sudden, resulting in stillbirth. Women undergoing expectant management of a preterm abruption should be hospitalized with immediate access to the delivery suite in case of acute decompensation.

UTERINE ATONY

The most common cause of hemorrhage is the failure of the uterus to contract after delivery of the placenta. Risk factors for uterine atony are well known, allowing anticipation of hemorrhage in many cases; however, they are only found in 50% of cases and are not typically predictive.[34] Conditions that overdistend the uterus, including macrosomia, polyhydramnios, and multiple gestations, lead to atony. Grand multiparity is a risk factor with Babinski and colleagues[35] and Fuchs and colleagues[36] both reporting an increased risk of atony with higher parity. Prolonged labor is a long-recognized risk factor and includes both inductions and augmentations. Retained placenta fragments can lead to atony and this is especially true if a succinate lobe is present. Inspection of the placenta after delivery should be routine and the uterine cavity explored if it looks incomplete. **Box 2** summarizes the common risk factors for hemorrhage.

> **Box 2**
> **Risk factors for uterine atony**
>
> - Overdistended uterus
>   - Macrosomia
>   - Multiple gestation
>   - Polyhydramnios
> - Prolonged labor
>   - Inductions
>   - Argumentations
> - Prolonged rupture of membranes
> - Grand multiparity
> - Retained placenta

The treatment of uterine atony is usually medical and consists of administration of oxytocic and/or prostaglandin derivatives (**Table 1**). In addition, bimanual compression is performed, a relatively easy technique that controls most uterine hemorrhage. In this technique, the posterior aspect of the uterine fundus is massaged through the abdomen while the anterior wall of the uterus is massaged through the vagina with the other hand. This should be done while medical treatment is being given. In addition to bimanual compression and medical management, resuscitation of the woman is critical. An effective circulating blood volume is essential for uterine perfusion and for the drugs administered to act on the myometrium. Without appropriate resuscitation, hypovolemic shock will develop and the atony will become persistent and ultimately irreversible. **Box 3** shows a typical algorithm for treating uterine atony.

VAGINAL AND CERVICAL LACERATION

Spontaneous delivery is associated with varying degrees of injury to the vagina and cervix that range from superficial to deep and very serious lacerations. The deeper lacerations of the vagina can involve the anal sphincter; extend into lateral vaginal

Table 1
Drugs commonly used in the treatment of postpartum atony

Drug Name	Dose	Route	Contraindication	Notes
Oxytocin	20–30 mg per 1 L of fluid	IV or IM	None	Should be initiated after delivery of the placenta
Ergot derivatives (methylergonovine)	0.2 mg	IM	Hypertension	IV administration can cause hypertensive crisis
Prostaglandin analogs F$_2\alpha$ – carboprost	0.25 mg	IM	Asthma	Side effects include diarrhea, fever, flushing less
Prostaglandin F$_2$	0.20 mg	Per rectum	None	effective than ergo or carboprost

Abbreviations. IM, intramuscular; IV, intravenous.

Box 3
Typical steps initiated for control of hemorrhage caused by uterine atony

1. Call for assistance
2. Initiate bimanual uterine compression
3. Confirm oxytocin is being administered
4. Start a second large-bore intravenous catheter for blood transfusions
5. Explore uterine cavity for retained placental fragments or lobes
6. Inspect the cervix and vagina for lacerations
7. Insert a Foley catheter to monitor urine output
8. Begin volume resuscitation and consider a blood transfusion

---

walls and even the ischiorectal fascia. It is of critical importance to recognize that bleeding after delivery while the uterus is contracted is suggestive of a genital tract laceration and/or retained placental fragments. Efforts to identify the source of the injury should be initiated immediately, as the bleeding may be brisk and can quickly lead to decompensation and shock.

CERVICAL LACERATION

The cervix is lacerated in up to 50% of normal vaginal deliveries.[37] Most of these are short, heal rapidly, and bleed minimally. Occasionally the tear will extend up into the lower uterine segment, uterine artery, and even extend retroperitoneally. These lacerations bleed profusely and repair may be quite difficult, even requiring a transabdominal approach in the most extreme cases. In general, the surgical repair of the cervical lacerations can be effected from the vagina with appropriate assistance, effective anesthesia, and vigorous resuscitation and blood replacement if necessary.

VAGINAL HEMATOMAS

Sometimes there is damage to the vaginal arteries, typically branches of the pudendal, and a hematoma occurs.[38] The incidence of puerperal hematoma varies from 1 in 300 to 1 in 1000 deliveries and the reported risk factors include nulliparity, episiotomy, and forceps delivery.[39,40] Usually the hematoma is small, does not expand, and will tamponade off. In more significant cases, the bleeding will result in an expanding hematoma that will develop rapidly, cause intense personal pain, and may dissect into the ischiorectal fascia and retroperitoneal spaces. Smaller nonexpanding hematomas may be managed expectantly; however, larger hematomas must be evacuated. Zahn and Yeomans[38] reported that half of women with a hematoma who require surgical intervention will also require a blood transfusion.

When incising and draining a hematoma, one should identify the point of maximal distension, open with a sharp scalpel, and evacuate the clot. If obvious, the bleeding artery should be identified and ligated, but often no obvious bleeding vessel is seen. In these cases, the cavity is closed in layers with hemostatic sutures placed and vaginal packing for 12 to 24 hours.

RESUSCITATION

The goal of resuscitation is to restore an effective circulating blood volume as efficiently as possible to avoid significant morbidity. Crystalloid solutions are typically used for initial volume resuscitation and are effective in cases of mild hemorrhage. The limitation of crystalloid resuscitation is due to reequilibration that results in only a proportion remaining in the intravascular circulation. Shoemaker and Kram[41] reported that only 20% of crystalloid remains in the circulation at 1 hour. Because of this reequilibration, initial crystalloid resuscitation typically occurs at 3 times the estimated blood loss. Depending on the degree of blood loss and crystalloid used, volume overload can be an issue after the initial event as the third spaced fluid returns to the intravascular space.

Colloid is sometimes used for resuscitation and even advocated by many as an alternative to crystalloid, as it is more likely to stay intravascular. A recent Cochrane analysis, however, has demonstrated a significant increase in cost but no benefit in patient outcome in critically ill nonpregnant patients.[42] The SAFE trial of 7000 nonrandomized nonpregnant patients reported similar results.[43]

With continued or massive hemorrhage, red blood cell transfusions will ultimately be required. Although the exact threshold at which replacement should be initiated has never been determined, most agree that a hematocrit (Hct) less than 21% to 25% in the face of ongoing hemorrhage is appropriate.[13] Although Morrison and colleagues[14] demonstrated that an Hct of between 18% and 25% is well tolerated in women who are isovolumic, but anemic, their conclusion drives home the point that interpretation of the Hct value is dependent on the likelihood of continued and ongoing blood loss. That is, an Hct of between 18% and 25% may be tolerated if there is no further bleeding.

Most cases of hemorrhage will require 1 to 2 units of red blood cells (RBCs) and the Hct can be expected to rise 3 to 4 volume percent per unit transfused. In large-volume hemorrhage, RBCs alone will not suffice and plasma and platelets will also be required depending on the amount of hemorrhage and the number of units of RBCs transfused. This need usually occurs in cases that require more than 4 to 8 units of RBCs. The ideal ratio of fresh frozen plasma to RBCs transfused in these cases has not been determined and higher ratios than have been traditionally used were recently recommended, based on data recently published.[44,45] In the face of this newer data, at least one large obstetric hospital has maintained a policy of transfusion of whole blood when available.[46] Platelets are usually required when levels fall below 50,000/μL and in patients experiencing massive transfusion (defined as 10 units of packed RBCs or more). Ideally, platelets obtained by apheresis from a single donor are transfused. When this is unavailable, which is often, random donor platelets are used and typically 5 to 6 donors are required to make "1" unit of platelets. A "unit" of platelets will usually raise the recipients' levels by 25,000 to 30,000.

Plasma is separated from whole blood immediately after donation and frozen for later use. When needed, it can be thawed in 30 minutes and is a source of all clotting factors, including fibrinogen. It should be given to correct clotting deficiencies related to large amounts of hemorrhage, as described previously. In addition, hemorrhage associated with a consumption coagulopathy, such as seen with abruption, typically requires plasma transfusion to increase fibrinogen levels if they fall to below 100 mg/dL. Cryoprecipitate is made from plasma and can be given if fibrinogen levels are very low and there is active oozing hemorrhage or oozing. It is particularly useful in cases in which volume overload is a concern. Transfusion-related acute lung injury (TRALI) has been described and is a life-threatening complication characterized by hypoxia, shortness of breath, and noncardiogenic pulmonary edema within 6 hours of transfusion and has been related to plasma infusion.[47] It is said to occur because of injury to the pulmonary capillaries, secondly to lipid products contained in stored blood components and may complicate 1 in 5000 cases. Alexander and colleagues[46] did not identify any cases in the 1540 women transfused in their study, suggesting that this complication is rare. The diagnosis of TRALI is very difficult to make, especially because its signs and symptoms are very similar to those seen with the volume overload sometimes encountered with those patients. When encountered, treatment is supportive.

Recombinant Activated Factor VIIa is a synthetic vitamin K–dependent protein that has been approved by the Food and Drug Administration for use in individuals with hemophilia. Recently, its use in surgery, trauma, and obstetrics has increased to control severe hemorrhage.[48,49] Recombinant Activated Factor VIIa, also known as NovoSeven, acts by binding to exposed tissue factor at the site of the tissue and vascular injury where it generates thrombin, which in turns activates platelets and the coagulation cascade. Thrombosis has been reported with the use of NovoSeven and when it occurs is usually seen with hemorrhage, not hemophilia cases.[48] Reports of thrombosis in obstetrics cases seem to be uncommon at this time.

SURGICAL MANAGEMENT OF HEMORRHAGE

Uterine atony is initially treated with pharmaceutical and resuscitative measures. When these are unsuccessful, or the hemorrhage is the result of a surgical injury, such as a uterine incision extension, surgical management is necessary. Uterine artery ligation, sometimes known as an O'Leary stitch, can be used, especially for uterine artery extensions. This stitch is placed through the lateral uterine wall and encompasses the uterine artery.

Uterine compression sutures were first described by B-Lynch and colleagues[50] in 1997. This technique and others like it compress the anterior and posterior walls of the bleeding uterus together.[50] In a follow-up to the previous report, B-Lynch[51] cited a failure rate of only 7 of 948 cases in which the technique was used. Although successful in many cases, there have been some case reports of ischemic necrosis with peritonitis.[52–54] At least one report exists of a defect in the uterine wall in a subsequent pregnancy after a B-Lynch and Cho stitch was performed.[55] Nevertheless, these compression sutures are relatively straightforward to perform, reported complications are isolated, and they may prevent a hysterectomy.

Uterine packing was used in the past to stop hemorrhage in women who desired to maintain their fertility, but fell out of favor because of concern over concealed hemorrhage and infection.[56] Newer techniques have been developed that minimize some of these concerns and include use of a Foley catheter and the Bakri balloon.[56] The Foley technique uses a 24F Foley catheter with a 30-mL balloon, which is inserted into the uterine cavity and filled with 60 to 80 mL of saline. This will compress the bleeding vessels, but the open tip also allows for drainage from the uterine cavity and monitoring of ongoing blood loss.

Angiographic embolization is sometimes resorted to when surgical access to bleeding vessels is difficult, such as in an intraperineal bleed. There are several studies reporting effectiveness with intractable hemorrhage and a 90% success rate. Although successful, pelvic embolization in the face of acute hemorrhage is logistically challenging and not always feasible. The patient may be too unstable for transport to the embolization laboratory and the interventional radiologist needed for the procedure may not be immediately available. Recently, prophylactic arterial catheter placement has been advocated for cases in which placenta percreta is likely. The increased accuracy of sonography in predicting these cases allows one to identify the women who are most likely to benefit. The prophylactic placement of the catheter allows for immediate embolization if heavy blood loss is encountered. Balloon-tipped catheters can be used as well and can be inflated when needed, as opposed to embolization being used. Complications of embolization are low, but include unexpected thrombosis and necrosis of the embolized tissue, leading to infection.

SUMMARY

Intrapartum hemorrhage is commonly encountered in obstetric practice. It can be brisk, resulting in large amounts of blood loss, quickly leading to shock, end-organ damage, and ultimately death. Intrapartum hemorrhage is included in this edition of the *Clinics* because it constitutes an emergency. Like any obstetric emergency, prompt recognition, identification of the cause, and timely intervention will result in excellent outcomes. Intrapartum hemorrhage is primarily caused by uterine atony, vaginal and cervical lacerations, uterine injury during cesarean delivery, and sometimes abruption. Management may include medical or surgical approaches or both and always requires adequate resuscitation with crystalloid and often transfusion of RBCs and other blood products. Learning to recognize the signs and symptoms of shock and familiarization with techniques for treatment and resuscitation are critical to a successful outcome.

REFERENCES

1. Loudon I. Deaths in childbed from the eighteenth century to 1935. Med Hist 1986; 30:1.
2. Chamberlain G. British maternal mortality in the 19th and early 20th centuries. J R Soc Med 2006;99:559.
3. Clark SL, Belfort MA, Dildy GA, et al. Maternal death in the 21st century: causes, prevention, and relationship to cesarean delivery. Am J Obstet Gynecol 2008; 199:36.e1.
4. Martin JA, Hamilton BE, Sutton PD, et al. Births: final data for 2003. Hyattsville, MD, National Center for Health Statistics. Natl Vital Stat Rep 2005;54(2):1–116.
5. Gerberding JL. Centers for Disease Control and Prevention: update: pregnancy-related mortality ratios, by year of death—United States, 1991–1999. MMWR Morb Mortal Wkly Rep 2003;52:1.
6. Lalonde A, Daviss BA, Acosta A, et al. Postpartum hemorrhage today: ICM/FIGO initiative 2004–2006. Int J Gynaecol Obstet 2006;94:243.
7. McCormick ML, Sanghvi HC, McIntosh N. Preventing postpartum hemorrhage in low-resource settings. Int J Gynaecol Obstet 2002;77:267.
8. The Joint Commission. Preventing maternal death, sentinel event alert. The Joint Commission; 2010. p. 44.
9. Silver RM, Landon MB, Rouse DJ, et al. Maternal morbidity associated with multiple repeat cesarean deliveries. Obstet Gynecol 2006;107:1226.
10. Edman CD, Toofanian A, MacDonald PC, et al. Placental clearance rate of maternal plasma androstenedione through placental estradiol formation: an indirect method of assessing uteroplacental blood flow. Am J Obstet Gynecol 1981; 141:1029.
11. Consensus Development Conference. Perioperative red cell transfusion, Vol. 7. Bethesda (MD): National Institutes of Health; 1988 (4).
12. Barbieri RL. Control of massive hemorrhage: lessons from Iraq reach the US labor and delivery suite. OBG Management 2007;19:8.
13. Hebert PC, Wells G, Blajchman MA, et al. A multicenter, randomized, controlled clinical trial of transfusion requirements in critical care. N Engl J Med 1999;340: 409.

14. Morrison JC, Martin RW, Dodson MK, et al. Blood transfusions after postpartum hemorrhage due to uterine atony. J Matern Fetal Investig 1991;1:209.
15. Pritchard JA. Changes in the blood volume during pregnancy and delivery. Anesthesiology 1965;26:393.
16. Zeeman GG, Cunningham FG, Pritchard JA. The magnitude of hemoconcentration with eclampsia. Hypertens Pregnancy 2009;28(2):127.
17. Pritchard JA, Baldwin RM, Dickey JC, et al. Blood volume changes in pregnancy and the puerperium, 2. Red blood cell loss and changes in apparent blood volume during and following vaginal delivery, cesarean section, and cesarean section plus total hysterectomy. Am J Obstet Gynecol 1962;84:1271.
18. Toledo P, McCarthy RJ, Hewlett BJ, et al. The accuracy of blood loss estimation after simulated vaginal delivery. Anesth Analg 2007;105:1736.
19. Sosa CG, Alathabe F, Belizan JM, et al. Risk factors for postpartum hemorrhage in vaginal deliveries in a Latin-American population. Obstet Gynecol 2009;113:1313.
20. Obstetrical hemorrhage. In: Cunningham FG, Leveno KJ, Bloom SL, et al, editors. Williams obstetrics. 23rd edition. New York: McGraw-Hill; 2010. p. 757.
21. Chang YL, Chang SD, Cheng PJ. Perinatal outcome in patients with placental abruption with and without antepartum hemorrhage. Int J Gynaecol Obstet 2001;75:193.
22. Pritchard JA, Brekken AL. Clinical and laboratory studies on severe abruptio placentae. Am J Obstet Gynecol 1967;97:681.
23. Bonnar J, McNicol GP, Douglas AS. The behavior of the coagulation and fibrinolytic mechanisms in abruptio placentae. J Obstet Gynaecol Br Commonw 1969;76:799.
24. Brame RG, Harbert GM Jr, McGaughey HS Jr, et al. Maternal risk in abruption. Obstet Gynecol 1968;31:224.
25. Salihu HM, Bekan B, Aliyu MH, et al. Perinatal mortality associated with abruptio placenta in singletons and multiples. Am J Obstet Gynecol 2005;193:198.
26. Cunningham FG, Hollier LM. Fetal death. In: Williams obstetrics. 20th edition. Norwalk (CT): Appleton & Lange; 1997:(Suppl 4).
27. Ananth CV, Berkowitz GS, Savitz DA, et al. Placental abruption and adverse perinatal outcomes. JAMA 1999;282:1646.
28. Ananth CV, Demissie K, Smulian JC, et al. Placenta previa in singleton and twin births in the United States, 1989 through 1998: a comparison of risk factor profiles and associated conditions. Am J Obstet Gynecol 2003;188:275.
29. Kramer MS, Usher RH, Pollack R, et al. Etiologic determinants of abruptio placentae. Obstet Gynecol 1997;89:221.
30. Kupferminc MJ, Eldor A, Steinman N, et al. Increased frequency of genetic thrombophilia in women with complications of pregnancy. N Engl J Med 1999;340:9.
31. Nath CA, Ananth CV, DeMarco C, et al. Low birthweight in relation to placental abruption and maternal thrombophilia status. Am J Obstet Gynecol 2008;198:293.e1.
32. Bond AL, Edersheim TG, Curry L, et al. Expectant management of abruptio placentae before 35 weeks gestation. Am J Perinatol 1989;6:121.
33. Elliott JP, Gilpin B, Strong TH Jr, et al. Chronic abruption—oligohydramnios sequence. J Reprod Med 1998;43:418.
34. Rouse DJ, MacPherson C, Landon M, et al. Blood transfusion and cesarean delivery. Obstet Gynecol 2006;108:891.
35. Babinszki A, Kerenyi T, Torok O, et al. Perinatal outcome in grand and great-grand multiparity: effects of parity on obstetric risk factors. Am J Obstet Gynecol 1999;181:669.

36. Fuchs K, Peretz BA, Marcovici R, et al. The "grand multipara"—is it a problem? A review of 5785 cases. Int J Gynaecol Obstet 1985;23:321.
37. Fahmy K, el-Gazar A, Sammour M, et al. Postpartum colposcopy of the cervix: injury and healing. Int J Gynaecol Obstet 1991;34:133.
38. Zahn CM, Yeomans ER. Postpartum hemorrhage: placenta accreta, uterine inversion and puerperal hematomas. Clin Obstet Gynecol 1990;33:422.
39. Propst AM, Thorp JM Jr. Traumatic vulvar hematomas: conservative versus surgical management. South Med J 1998;91:144.
40. Cunningham FG. Genital tract lacerations and puerperal hematomas. In: Gilstrap LC III, Cunningham FG, Van Dorsten JP, editors. Operative obstetrics. 2nd edition. New York: McGraw-Hill; 2002. p. 223.
41. Shoemaker WC, Kram HB. Comparison of the effects of crystalloids and colloids on hemodynamic oxygen transport, mortality and morbidity. In: Simmons RS, Udeko AJ, editors. Debates in general surgery. Chicago: Year Book; 1991.
42. Perel P, Roberts I. Colloids versus crystalloids for fluid resuscitation in critically ill patients. Cochrane Database Syst Rev 2007;(4):CD000567.
43. Finfer S, Bellomo R, Boyce N, et al. A comparison of albumin and saline for fluid resuscitation in the intensive care unit. N Engl J Med 2004;350:2247.
44. Laine E, Steadman R, Calhoun L, et al. Comparison of RBCs and FFP with whole blood during liver transplant surgery. Transfusion 2003;43:322.
45. Spinella PC, Perkins JC, Grathwohl KW, et al. Fresh whole blood transfusions in coalition military, foreign national, and enemy combatant patients during Operation Iraqi Freedom at a US combat support hospital. World J Surg 2008;32:2.
46. Alexander JM, Sarode R, McIntire DD, et al. Use of whole blood in the management of hypovolemia due to obstetric hemorrhage. Obstet Gynecol 2009;113:1320.
47. Silliman CC, Boshkov LK, Mehdizadehkashi Z, et al. Transfusion-related acute lung injury: epidemiology and a prospective analysis of etiologic factors. Blood 2003;101:454.
48. Mannucci PM, Levi M. Prevention and treatment of major blood loss. N Engl J Med 2007;356:2301.
49. Franchini M, Lippi G, Franchi M. The use of recombinant activated factor VII in obstetric and gynaecological haemorrhage. BJOG 2007;114:8.
50. B-Lynch CB, Coker A, Laval AH, et al. The B-Lynch surgical technique for control of massive postpartum hemorrhage: an alterative to hysterectomy? Five cases reported. Br J Obstet Gynaecol 1997;104:372.
51. B-Lynch C. Partial ischemic necrosis of the uterus following a uterine brace compression suture. BJOG 2005;112:126.
52. Gottlieb AG, Pandipati S, Davis KM, et al. Uterine necrosis. A complication of uterine compression sutures. Obstet Gynecol 2008;112:429.
53. Joshi VM, Shrivastava M. Partial ischemic necrosis of the uterus following a uterine brace compression suture. BJOG 2004;111:279.
54. Ochoa M, Allaire AD, Stitely ML. Pyometria after hemostatic square suture technique. Obstet Gynecol 2002;99:506.
55. Akoury H, Sherman C. Uterine wall partial thickness necrosis following combined B-Lynch and Cho square sutures for the treatment of primary postpartum hemorrhage. J Obstet Gynaecol Can 2008;30:421.
56. Hsu S, Rodgers B, Lele A, et al. Use of packing in obstetric hemorrhage of uterine origin. J Reprod Med 2003;48:69.

Pulmonary Embolism and Amniotic Fluid Embolism in Pregnancy

Matthew C. Brennan, MD, Lisa E. Moore, MD*

KEYWORDS

- Pulmonary embolus • Amniotic fluid embolus • Venous thrombosis

KEY POINTS

- A suspected pulmonary embolism or amniotic fluid embolism (AFE) constitutes an obstetric emergency.
- There are many changes occurring during pregnancy and postpartum that play a role in the increase in clot formation.
- Early initiation of treatment is the greatest factor in survival.
- There are no diagnostic tests with demonstrated accuracy for AFE.

INTRODUCTION

Pulmonary thromboembolism and AFE make up 2 of the most common causes of maternal death in the United States, together accounting for almost 23% of maternal death.[1] A recent study evaluated 95 maternal deaths of 1.4 million pregnancies over a 6-year period in the United States[1] and found that pulmonary thromboembolism and AFE were 2 of the most commonly seen causes of maternal death. AFE accounted for 14% of the total maternal deaths, and pulmonary thromboembolism accounted for 9% of the maternal deaths. Any discussion regarding obstetric emergencies requires a thorough understanding of these 2 entities. This article reviews the diagnosis and management of AFE and pulmonary thromboembolism in pregnancy.

PULMONARY THROMBOEMBOLISM

Pulmonary embolism and venous thrombosis represent one of the more common life-threatening emergencies faced by obstetric providers. Improved assessment of risks

---

Division of Maternal Fetal Medicine, Department of Obstetrics and Gynecology, School of Medicine, University of New Mexico, MSC 10 5580, 1 University of New Mexico, Albuquerque, NM 87131-0001, USA
* Corresponding author.
E-mail address: Lemoore@salud.unm.edu

Obstet Gynecol Clin N Am 40 (2013) 27–35
http://dx.doi.org/10.1016/j.ogc.2012.11.005
0889-8545/13/$ – see front matter © 2013 Elsevier Inc. All rights reserved.

and institution of appropriate thromboprophylaxis has led to improvement, but venous thromboembolism remains a leading cause of maternal mortality in the developing world, including the United States.[1,2] The incidence of pregnancy-related venous thromboembolism has been reported to be as high as 1.72 per 1000 deliveries, and the incidence of pulmonary embolism in pregnancy is 200 per 100,000 woman-years.[3] Thromboembolism usually presents unprovoked and with little warning, therefore rapid diagnosis and treatment is critical to preventing maternal deaths. An understanding of the risk factors, clinical symptoms, diagnostic testing, and treatment modalities is necessary to make a rapid diagnosis and institute timely therapy.

Risk Factors

Pregnancy is a hypercoaguable state and is in itself a risk factor for thrombosis. The relative risk for venous thromboembolism among pregnant and postpartum women is 4.29.[3] Venous thromboembolism can occur at any point in pregnancy or postpartum, although half of pregnancy-related venous thromboembolism occurs in the postpartum period.[4] It is therefore important to maintain a heightened suspicion for thromboembolism, and prevention should be an aspect of all postpartum care.

There are many changes occurring during pregnancy and postpartum that play a role in the increase in clot formation, including

- Hypercoagulability
- Decreased mobility
- Venous stasis

Pregnancy is a state of relative hypercoagulability with an increase in levels of fibrinogen; factors VIII, IX, and X; von Willebrand factor; and plasma activator inhibitors 1 and 2.[5] Women may have decreased mobility in labor because of pain, epidural anesthesia, and fetal monitoring. Women undergoing cesarean delivery are especially at risk and carry twice the risk of venous thromboembolism. The American College of Obstetricians and Gynecologists recommends that all women undergoing cesarean delivery have pneumatic compression devices placed before cesarean delivery and that women with additional risk factors may require thromboprophylaxis with heparin.[5]

Certain medical conditions carry an increased risk of venous thromboembolism. Among these conditions, having a personal history of a known thrombophilia carries the greatest risk with an odds ratio of 52.[4] Other risk factors for thromboembolism include[5–8]

- Personal history of venous thrombosis
- Antiphospholipid antibody syndrome
- Lupus
- Heart disease
- Sickle cell disease
- Black race
- Advanced maternal age
- Diabetes
- Obesity
- Operative delivery
- Smoking
- Hypertension

Stratifying women based on risk factors may help to determine who needs thromboprophylaxis in pregnancy and in what situations. Several groups have evaluated weighted scoring systems to guide thromboprophylaxis in high risk pregnant women.[9–11] Further study in this area may allow us to better stratify women based on risk and offer proper and safe prevention strategies.

Diagnosis

Treatment success of pulmonary thromboembolism relies on immediate institution of therapy, which requires a heightened awareness of symptoms. Recognition of symptoms of pulmonary thromboembolism is difficult because many of the symptoms women complain of in pulmonary embolism are frequent complaints among normal pregnant women and are often overlooked by providers. Also complicating making a rapid diagnosis is that up to 86% of thromboembolism occurs in women with no previous history of venous thromboembolism.[12] In nonpregnant patients, dyspnea or tachypnea was present in 90% of cases of acute pulmonary embolism.[13] Shortness of breath is a common complaint among pregnant women and is therefore not a reliable indicator of women with pulmonary embolism in pregnancy.

In the setting of fatal pulmonary embolism, 65% of the fatalities occur in the first hour after onset of symptoms.[14] Because of the risk of sudden death with pulmonary thromboembolism, treatment should not be delayed for diagnostic testing if there is a high clinical suspicion of pulmonary embolus. Anticoagulation should be instituted immediately in any pregnant woman who complains of acute onset of shortness of breath and in whom pulmonary embolism is of concern. There are multiple primary and ancillary testing methods available in clinical practice for the evaluation of shortness of breath, including electrocardiogram (ECG), chest radiograph, arterial blood gas, ventilation-perfusion (VQ) scan, and computed tomography (CT). Evaluation of venous thrombosis in pregnancy requires the clinician to balance the fetal and maternal risk of radiation exposure, availability of testing in local institutions, quickness of available testing, and accuracy of testing methods.

Approximately 80% of women with a pulmonary embolism have evidence of a deep venous thrombosis (DVT). For this reason, pregnant women who are suspected of having a pulmonary embolism and have signs or symptoms of a DVT should undergo evaluation of the lower extremities.[15] Compression ultrasonography of the lower extremities is the modality of choice in the evaluation of DVT in pregnant women. If a DVT is found on evaluation, anticoagulation therapy should be instituted before any further evaluation.

In pregnant women who are suspected of having a pulmonary embolism and who do not have signs or symptoms of DVT, the evaluation should start with ruling out pulmonary embolism and not with DVT evaluation. In nonpregnant patients, CT has been shown to be superior in the diagnosis of pulmonary embolism.[16] This study did not include pregnant women and the optimal choice for initial evaluation of pulmonary embolism in pregnancy is not known. One method that can be used in deciding between CT and VQ scan is to start with a chest radiograph. A recent study found that chest radiograph can be used to determine whether to proceed with a CT scan or a VQ scan.[17] If the result of the initial chest radiograph is normal, then VQ scan may be more likely to yield a diagnostic result than a CT scan. **Fig. 1** shows an algorithm for evaluation of suspected pulmonary embolism in pregnancy. Guidelines from the American Thoracic Society recommend that the evaluation of pulmonary embolism in pregnant women starts with a chest radiograph as the discriminatory test.[15] If the result of this radiograph is normal, the recommendation is to proceed with VQ scan. If the result of the initial chest radiograph is abnormal, the recommendation is to proceed with a CT scan. One difficulty that frequently arises with this algorithm is the availability of these tests in local institutions. CT has widely replaced VQ scan in the evaluation of pulmonary embolism in nonpregnant patients, and therefore, the availability of VQ scan may

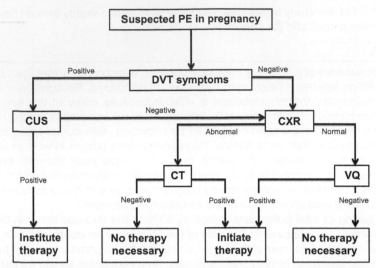

Fig. 1. CUS, compression ultrasound; CXR, chest radiograph; DVT, deep venous thrombosis; PE, pulmonary embolism.

be limited. Knowing the availability of these modalities in each institution is important when deciding which method to choose in the evaluation of a pregnant patient with acute signs and symptoms of pulmonary embolus.

Treatment

Pulmonary embolism is an acute event that can lead to devastating consequences. In general, treatment of thromboembolism is safe and readily available in most centers. Treatment should therefore not be withheld for diagnostic testing if clinical suspicion is high. Anticoagulation with unfractionated heparin (UFH), low-molecular-weight heparin (LMWH), and warfarin are the main treatments of thromboembolism in pregnancy and the postpartum period.

Heparins are considered the mainstay of treatment of thromboembolic disease in pregnancy. Warfarin freely crosses the placenta, and its use in pregnancy is associated with teratogenicity and an increased risk of bleeding in the fetus.[18] It is therefore not routinely used as an anticoagulant in pregnant women. Both UFH and LMWH do not cross the placenta and therefore pose very little risk to the fetus. Although LMWH and UFH are both effective and relatively safe in pregnancy, there is limited information available to determine which of these should be primarily used in pregnancy. In nonpregnant patients, a Cochrane review found LMWH to be more effective than UFH for the initial treatment of venous thromboembolism while also leading to a decrease in major hemorrhage.[19] Both medications have advantages and disadvantages that must be balanced when choosing an initial treatment of thromboembolism in pregnancy.

When compared with LMWH, UFH is less expensive and has a shorter half-life. The shorter half-life of UFH may allow for the use of regional anesthesia in labor and may decrease the risk of significant peripartum bleeding. Also, it is possible to determine the anticoagulant effect of UFH by measuring the partial thromboplastin time and reverse with protamine if needed. The American Society of Regional Anesthesia and

Pain Medicine recommend delaying catheter placement for 24 hours after the last therapeutic dose of LMWH.[20] A few advantages of LMWH include decreased risk of heparin-induced thrombocytopenia, longer half-life, easier dosing, more predictable therapeutic response, less bruising at injection sites, fewer episodes of major bleeding, and ease of monitoring.[19,21]

The choice for initial therapy of an acute thromboembolic event in pregnancy is LMWH or UFH given intramuscularly. Outpatient treatment is appropriate in most instances. Settings in which inpatient treatment with intravenous heparin is appropriate are cases of large pulmonary embolism in an unstable patient or an actively laboring patient. Although both LMWH and UFH are recommended treatment options, LMWH is the recommended treatment in pregnant patients with an acute pulmonary embolism by the American College of Chest Physicians.[22] Following are the recommended options for treatment of acute pulmonary embolism in pregnancy:

- UFH given subcutaneously every 12 hours in doses adjusted to target activated partial thromboplastin time in the therapeutic range (1.5–2.5, midinterval)
- Weight-adjusted full treatment dose of LMWH
  - Enoxaparin 1 mg/kg every 12 hours
  - Dalteparin 200 units/kg once daily
  - Tinzaparin 175 units/kg once daily
  - Dalteparin 100 units/kg every 12 hours

There are 2 recommended methods for anticoagulation at term in anticipation of labor. One method is to switch from LMWH to UFH in the last month of pregnancy. Based on the shorter half-life of UFH, women may continue their anticoagulation up to the onset of labor and may have the option to undergo regional anesthesia. The alternative method is to continue LMWH and then discontinue 24 hours before induction of labor or planned cesarean delivery.

There are limited data available, but postpartum anticoagulation should be restarted no sooner than 4 to 6 hours after a vaginal delivery and 6 to 12 hours after a cesarean delivery.[5] Anticoagulation therapy should then be continued for 6 weeks postpartum.[22] Warfarin, UFH, and LMWH are all considered safe in breastfeeding mothers. Postpartum anticoagulation options are

- Warfarin with a target international normalized ratio of 2.0 to3.0, with initial overlap of UFH or LMWH
- Prophylactic LMWH

AMNIOTIC FLUID EMBOLISM

The passage of amniotic fluid into the maternal circulation may cause a life-threatening cascade of events including respiratory and cardiovascular arrest and multisystem organ failure. This event, known as AFE, occurs in 1 in 8000 to 1 in 80,000 deliveries.[23,24]

As a clinical entity, AFE was first described by Steiner and Lushbaugh[25] in 1941. Clark and colleagues[26] have established a national registry for AFE. Based on the data contained therein, Clark has suggested that the events are more accurately characterized as anaphylaxis and has suggested the term anaphylactoid syndrome of pregnancy.

AFE typically occurs during labor and delivery but has been described up to 48 hours postpartum. AFE has been described during abortion, amnioinfusion, amniocentesis, after removal of cerclage, during manual removal of the placenta, and after blunt abdominal trauma.[23,27,28]

Risk Factors

Using the Healthcare Cost and Utilization Project Nationwide Inpatient Sample (NIS) database, records were extracted that included an ICD-9 (international Classification of Disease 9th revision) code for AFE.[24] Each identified case was then reviewed for procedures consistent with a clinical diagnosis of AFE. Of 2,940,360 records, 227 had a discharge diagnosis of AFE. Analysis indicated that maternal age of 35 years or more, black race, placenta previa, preeclampsia, cesarean delivery, and forceps or vacuum delivery were strongly associated with the occurrence of AFE. Age less than 20 years seemed to have a protective effect. No difference was found between rural or urban teaching and urban nonteaching hospitals in the rate of occurrence. A limitation of this study was that it was impossible to determine whether AFE occurred due to operative procedures (ie, cesarean or forceps/vacuum delivery) or conversely, whether operative procedures were performed because the patient was in distress from an AFE.

A second important study abstracted data from the United States via the Pregnancy Mortality Surveillance System (PMSS) of the CDC, from the United Kingdom using the Confidential Enquiries into Maternal Deaths between 2003 and 2008, from Canada using the Discharge Abstract Database of the Canadian Institute for Health, from the Netherlands, and from Australia.[29] The only factors that were consistently associated with AFE across the 5 countries were maternal age and induction of labor.

Pathophysiology

The pathophysiology of AFE is an area of controversy. It is presumed that amniotic fluid enters the maternal circulation. Paradoxically, AFE has been described up to 48 hours postpartum. It has been proposed that amniotic fluid and fetal debris may be trapped in the uterine veins and released into the circulation during uterine involution. Attempts to re-create the syndrome in animal models by injecting amniotic fluid directly into the circulation using goats, monkeys, and rabbits have been largely unsuccessful.[23,30] Fetal squamous cells have been found in the circulation of women who do not experience AFE, and conversely, AFE has been diagnosed in women in whom fetal cells and debris were not present postmortem. Clark and colleagues[26,31] theorize that amniotic fluid contains vasoactive elements including bradykinin, thromboxane, leukotrienes, and arachidonic metabolites. When these substances enter the maternal circulation, even in small amounts, they may trigger an immunologic response resulting in AFE. Serum tryptase, urinary histamine, and serum complement levels were measured in 9 women with a diagnosis of AFE compared with 22 women in a control group. Tryptase and histamine are products of mast cell degranulation indicating an immune response. Tests for serum tryptase and urinary histamine gave negative results in all 9 women. However, all women with AFE had abnormally low levels of complement.[32,33]

Clinical Manifestations

Clinically, any combination of sudden cardiovascular collapse, dyspnea or respiratory arrest, altered mental status, systemic hypotension, cyanosis, and hemorrhage are consistent with AFE. In the AFE registry, hypotension and nonreassuring fetal status were the common presentations. Respiratory distress (93%), cardiac arrest (87%), and coagulopathy (83%) were also seen.[26]

Diagnosis

The diagnosis of AFE is clinical and exclusionary. AFE should be suspected during pregnancy or up to 48 hours postpartum in women who develop hypotension, respiratory or cardiovascular collapse, DIC (disseminated intravascular coagulation), coma, and/or seizures in the absence of other identifiable causes. Laboratory tests are not specific.

Management

Early recognition is the most important factor associated with a positive maternal outcome. Management is supportive. There are no proven accepted therapies. If undelivered, delivery of the fetus and placenta should be expedited. Immediate resuscitation should be undertaken with placement of intravenous lines, continuous cardiac monitoring, and serial determinations of coagulation values. The ECG may show signs of right ventricular strain with tachycardia. Uterine atony and postpartum hemorrhage with disseminated intravascular coagulation should be anticipated, and a massive transfusion protocol should be initiated. Intubation should be available if needed. Pressors may be required to treat hypotension.

Morbidity and Mortality

Because there is no specific criterion for diagnosing an AFE, morbidity and mortality statistics may not be accurate. In the US national registry, Clark reported a 15% maternal intact survival rate and 61% mortality with 36% dying in the first 2 hours. Fetal mortality was 21%, although 50% of the survivors had permanent neurologic injury.[26] More recent population-based studies suggest that maternal mortality from AFE may be between 13% and 26.4%.[24]

SUMMARY

A suspected pulmonary embolism or AFE constitutes an obstetric emergency. In women with suspected pulmonary embolism, the evaluation should start with chest radiograph as a discriminator and then proceed with a VQ scan if the result of the chest radiograph is normal or with a CT scan if the result is abnormal. Therapeutic anticoagulation with LMWH or UFH is the treatment of choice in women with a pulmonary embolism in pregnancy, although the decision on which medication to use should be individualized. AFE may be more similar to an anaphylactoid reaction than to an embolic event. The diagnosis of AFE is one of exclusion. There are no diagnostic tests with demonstrated accuracy. Postmortem, the presence of fetal cells and debris in the pulmonary vasculature is considered diagnostic; however, the absence of fetal cells or debris does not rule out the diagnosis. Early initiation of treatment is the greatest factor in survival. Management of AFE is supportive because there are no proven therapies.

REFERENCES

1. Clark SL, Belfort MA, Dildy GA, et al. Maternal death in the 21st century: causes, prevention, and relationship to cesarean delivery. Am J Obstet Gynecol 2008; 199(1):36.e1–5 [discussion: 91–2.e7–11].
2. Chang J, Elam-Evans LD, Berg CJ, et al. Pregnancy-related mortality surveillance-United States, 1991-99. MMWR Surveill Summ 2003;52(2):1–8.
3. Heit JA, Kobbervig CE, James AH, et al. Trends in the incidence of venous thromboembolism during pregnancy or postpartum: a 30-year population-based study. Ann Intern Med 2005;143(10):697–706.
4. James AH, Jamison MG, Brancazio LR, et al. Venous thromboembolism during pregnancy and the postpartum period: incidence, risk factors, and mortality. Am J Obstet Gynecol 2006;194(5):1311–5.

5. James A. Practice bulletin no. 123: thromboembolism in pregnancy. Obstet Gynecol 2011;118(3):718–29.
6. Knight M. Antenatal pulmonary embolism: risk factors, management and outcomes. BJOG 2008;115(4):453–61.
7. Larsen TB, Sorensen HT, Gislum M, et al. Maternal smoking, obesity, and risk of venous thromboembolism during pregnancy and the puerperium: a population-based nested case-control study. Thromb Res 2007;120(4):505–9.
8. Morgan ES, Wilson E, Watkins T, et al. Maternal obesity and venous thromboembolism. Int J Obstet Anesth 2012;21(3):253–63.
9. Schoenbeck D, Nicolle A, Newbegin K, et al. The use of a scoring system to guide thromboprophylaxis in a high-risk pregnant population. Thrombosis 2011;2011: 652796.
10. Cavazza S, Rainaldi MP, Adduci A, et al. Thromboprophylaxis following cesarean delivery: one site prospective pilot study to evaluate the application of a risk score model. Thromb Res 2012;129(1):28–31.
11. Bauersachs RM, Dudenhausen J, Faridi A, et al. Risk stratification and heparin prophylaxis to prevent venous thromboembolism in pregnant women. Thromb Haemost 2007;98(6):1237–45.
12. Gherman RB, Goodwin TM, Leung B, et al. Incidence, clinical characteristics, and timing of objectively diagnosed venous thromboembolism during pregnancy. Obstet Gynecol 1999;94(5 Pt 1):730–4.
13. Stein PD, Terrin ML, Hales CA, et al. Clinical, laboratory, roentgenographic, and electrocardiographic findings in patients with acute pulmonary embolism and no pre-existing cardiac or pulmonary disease. Chest 1991;100(3):598–603.
14. Stein PD, Henry JW. Prevalence of acute pulmonary embolism among patients in a general hospital and at autopsy. Chest 1995;108(4):978–81.
15. Leung AN, Bull TM, Jaeschke R, et al. American Thoracic Society documents: an official American Thoracic Society/Society of Thoracic Radiology Clinical Practice Guideline–Evaluation of Suspected Pulmonary Embolism in Pregnancy. Radiology 2012;262(2):635–46.
16. Stein PD, Fowler SE, Goodman LR, et al. Multidetector computed tomography for acute pulmonary embolism. N Engl J Med 2006;354(22):2317–27.
17. Cahill AG, Stout MJ, Macones GA, et al. Diagnosing pulmonary embolism in pregnancy using computed-tomographic angiography or ventilation-perfusion. Obstet Gynecol 2009;114(1):124–9.
18. Stevenson RE, Burton OM, Ferlauto GJ, et al. Hazards of oral anticoagulants during pregnancy. JAMA 1980;243(15):1549–51.
19. van Dongen CJ, van den Belt AG, Prins MH, et al. Fixed dose subcutaneous low molecular weight heparins versus adjusted dose unfractionated heparin for venous thromboembolism. Cochrane Database Syst Rev 2004;(4):CD001100.
20. Horlocker TT. Regional anaesthesia in the patient receiving antithrombotic and antiplatelet therapy. Br J Anaesth 2011;107(Suppl 1):i96–106.
21. Greer IA, Nelson-Piercy C. Low-molecular-weight heparins for thromboprophylaxis and treatment of venous thromboembolism in pregnancy: a systematic review of safety and efficacy. Blood 2005;106(2):401–7.
22. Bates SM, Greer IA, Pabinger I, et al. Venous thromboembolism, thrombophilia, antithrombotic therapy, and pregnancy: American College of Chest Physicians Evidence-Based Clinical Practice Guidelines (8th edition). Chest 2008; 133(Suppl 6):844S–86S.
23. Gist RS, Stafford IP, Leibowitz AB, et al. Amniotic fluid embolism. Anesth Analg 2009;108(5):1599–602.

24. Abenhaim HA, Azoulay L, Kramer MS, et al. Incidence and risk factors of amniotic fluid embolisms: a population-based study on 3 million births in the United States. Am J Obstet Gynecol 2008;199(1):49.e1–8.
25. Steiner PE, Lushbaugh CC. Maternal pulmonary embolism by amniotic fluid - as a cause of obstetric shock and unexpected deaths in obstetrics. JAMA 1941;117: 1245.
26. Clark SL, Hankins GD, Dudley DA, et al. Amniotic fluid embolism: analysis of the national registry. Am J Obstet Gynecol 1995;172(4 Pt 1):1158–67 [discussion: 1167–9].
27. Conde-Agudelo A, Romero R. Amniotic fluid embolism: an evidence-based review. Am J Obstet Gynecol 2009;201(5):445.e1–13.
28. Haines J, Wilkes RG. Non-fatal amniotic fluid embolism after cervical suture removal. Br J Anaesth 2003;90(2):244–7.
29. Knight M, Berg C, Brocklehurst P, et al. Amniotic fluid embolism incidence, risk factors and outcomes: a review and recommendations. BMC Pregnancy Childbirth 2012;12:17.
30. Spence M, Mason KG. Experimental amniotic fluid embolism in rabbits. Am J Obstet Gynecol 1974;119(8):1073–8.
31. Clarke J, Butt M. Maternal collapse. Curr Opin Obstet Gynecol 2005;17(2): 157–60.
32. Benson MD, Kobayashi H, Silver RK, et al. Immunologic studies in presumed amniotic fluid embolism. Obstet Gynecol 2001;97(4):510–4.
33. Benson MD, Lindberg RE. Amniotic fluid embolism, anaphylaxis, and tryptase. Am J Obstet Gynecol 1996;175(3 Pt 1):737.

Emergency Cesarean Delivery
Special Precautions

Joey E. Tyner, MD*, William F. Rayburn, MD, MBA

KEYWORDS

- Cesarean delivery • Emergency • Operative obstetrics • Special precautions

KEY POINTS

- Precautions preoperatively, introperatively, and postpartum are paramount to reduce morbidity and mortality.
- The decision-to-delivery interval for an emergency cesarean delivery is arbitrary but must be as rapid and safe as possible.
- Periodic simulation drills are valuable to improve teamwork readiness and enhance communication skills.

INTRODUCTION

An emergent cesarean delivery is performed to immediately improve maternal or fetal outcomes for such indications as fetal distress, prolapsed cord, maternal hemorrhage from previa or trauma, uterine rupture, and complete placental abruption.[1] In contrast, an urgent cesarean delivery is performed for maternal or fetal compromise, which is not immediately life-threatening. Compared with scheduled surgery, an emergency cesarean is associated with increased risks of severe hemorrhage, anesthetic complications from rapid administration of general anesthesia, and accidental injury to the fetus or nearby abdominopelvic organs.

In the United States, more than 1 million cesarean deliveries are performed annually, accounting for 33% of births in 2009 compared with 15% worldwide. Since 1996, this rate has increased by more than 50%.[2] Bergholt and colleagues[3] reported an incidence of emergency cesarean delivery to be 7.2% in a low-risk population, and Haerskjold and colleagues[4] reported a similar rate at 8.7%.

It is paramount to prepare for emergent cesarean delivery to reduce morbidity and mortality. This article reviews special precautions to be undertaken before, during, and after an emergent cesarean delivery, and reflects recent publications in peer-review medical journals.

Division of Maternal Fetal Medicine, Department of Obstetrics and Gynecology, University of New Mexico School of Medicine, MSC 10 5580, 1 University of New Mexico, Albuquerque, NM 87131-0001, USA
* Corresponding author.
E-mail address: jtyner@salud.unm.edu

Obstet Gynecol Clin N Am 40 (2013) 37–45
http://dx.doi.org/10.1016/j.ogc.2012.11.003
0889-8545/13/$ – see front matter © 2013 Elsevier Inc. All rights reserved.

obgyn.theclinics.com

DECISION TO DELIVERY

The decision-to-delivery interval for an emergency cesarean delivery is the time in minutes from the decision to undertake surgery until delivery of the infant. The standard that is currently accepted by the American College of Obstetricians and Gynecologists, the Royal College of Obstetricians and Gynecologists, and the American Academy of Pediatrics is within 30 minutes.[5] This guideline is greatly disputed, because it has been claimed that that an interval greater than 30 minutes was not necessarily associated with increased neonatal morbidity or mortality.[6,7] Thomas and colleagues[1] propose an interval of 75 minutes as the threshold for causing worsened maternal and fetal outcomes, but admit that adoption of a more prolonged time could lead to complacency. Regardless of time, every effort must be made to proceed as rapidly and safely as possible. Accomplishing this is determined by the availability of facilities and staff, the performance and interpretation of fetal monitoring, and the decision-making practices.[8,9]

In 2009, Leung and colleagues[10] correlated deterioration of cord arterial pH with prolonged delivery time when the underlying cause of fetal distress was irreversible. When the cause was reversible, such an association was not present.[11] Conditions listed as being irreversible included placental abruption, cord prolapse, uterine rupture, preeclampsia, and failed instrumental delivery. Reversible conditions include iatrogenic uterine hyperstimulation, hypotension following regional anesthesia, aortocaval compression, and after external cephalic version. According to their report, with the irreversible conditions, a call for a decision-to-delivery interval of less than 30 minutes was proposed because they achieved a median value of 10 minutes.

PREOPERATIVE PRECAUTIONS
Informed Consent

The United States is recognized as the country of modern informed consent, in which the patient is engaged in decision making.[12] Physicians are required by law and medical ethics to obtain the informed consent of their patients before performing any surgery.[13] After deciding to undergo an emergency cesarean delivery, the obstetrician should at least obtain verbal informed consent. In rare cases in which informed consent is not possible (eg, maternal cardiac arrest), the physician may proceed with emergency cesarean delivery with a recommended initiation ideally after 4 minutes of maternal cardiac arrest.[14] This can be difficult to achieve despite drills and simulations, and consideration should be made to store emergency delivery equipment in the resuscitation cart.[15]

Antibiotic Prophylaxis

The ACOG Committee on Obstetric Practice recommends antibiotic prophylaxis for all cesarean deliveries unless it is not possible. For these emergencies, antibiotics should be administered as soon as safely possible.[16] Antibiotic prophylaxis has proved to be beneficial to reduce the risk of postoperative infection including endometritis and wound infection. In 2002, the Cochrane Library reported reductions in endometritis (60%–70%) and wound infection (30%–65%) with the use of prophylactic antibiotics.[11]

Allergies should be considered. Penicillin anaphylaxis is estimated to occur in 1 in 2500 to 25,000 patients.[17] During an emergency situation, it may be beneficial to have alternatives for antibiotic prophylaxis (for patients with a penicillin allergy) posted in the operating room. For women with a serious allergy to penicillin (immediate hypersensitivity reaction), a prophylactic regimen of metronidazole (500 mg) or clindamycin (900 mg) should be administered intravenously in combination with 1.5 mg/kg of gentamicin.[18] For women with a mild allergy to penicillin, a cephalosporin may be administered. By performing skin testing well in advance, risk may be determined while searching for clinical features and the elapsed time of the reaction.[19]

Obesity

The prevalence of obesity in the United States has increased greatly, and obese women are at greater risk for pregnancy complications, including difficulty in performing an emergent cesarean delivery. In the United States, the estimated prevalence for obesity among pregnant women varies from 18.5% to 35.3%.[20] Obese patients are more likely to have wound breakdowns, infections, venous thromboembolism, preeclampsia, and gestational diabetes.[21] In addition, higher prepregnancy body mass index is a risk factor for morbidity from obstetric anesthesia. There are higher rates of difficult airways and failed intubations in the obese patient.[22] Special resources may be necessary, such as blood products, a large operating table, appropriately sized blood pressure cuffs, and sequential compression devices for the delivery.

Time-out

In 2004, the Joint Commission mandated a standardized time-out (universal protocol) at the initiation of every surgical procedure.[23] Conley and coauthors emphasized the use of time-outs especially before emergency surgeries.[24] A time-out can be performed expeditiously and allows all team members to coordinate their care. Listed in **Box 1** is our institution's time-out protocol for all cesarean deliveries, which we have used successfully for every cesarean delivery during this past year.

Anesthesia

The choice of regional or general anesthesia is influenced by factors such as preexisting epidural anesthesia, urgency of the procedure, maternal status, physician and patient preference, and safety. For elective cesarean delivery, central neuraxial blockade is

---

Box 1
Time-out checklist used at the University of New Mexico for all cesarean deliveries

1. Surgeon: "Can we begin the time-out?"

   Team introductions as needed.

2. Surgeon: situation, background, assessment, recommendation (SBAR) report to team.

   SBAR will be updated as needed.

3. Registered Nurse (RN) Circulator: confirm patient. "This is ___, her date of birth/medical record number is ___."

   Anesthesiology: "That is correct."

4. Anesthesiology: allergies, antibiotics.

5. RN Circulator: confirm with scrub technician and surgeons. Verify that all supplies/equipment/consents, and so forth present.

   "Do we have everything we need?"

6. Surgeon: share any special instructions.

   "Any concerns?"

   "I expect you to speak up if there are any questions or concerns."

7. Surgeon: "Time-out is complete."

most commonly administered. However, under severe time constraints, as in emergency cesarean delivery, general anesthesia is frequently administered.[25,26] Potential complications of general anesthesia are failed intubation, maternal pulmonary aspiration of gastric contents, uterine atony and excess hemorrhage, and neonatal depression.[27]

Urethral Catheter Placement

To prevent bladder distention and thus obstruction of the lower uterine segment, urethral catheters are placed before cesarean delivery. There is no strong evidence that this practice is advantageous and it may be necessary to bypass catheter placement in emergent situations. In 2011, Li and colleagues[28] reported decreased urinary tract infections and no increase of urinary retention or intraoperative difficulties with omission of the ureteral catheter. Omitting a Foley catheter placement with special care to avoid the bladder can be achieved with minimal complications.[29] An alternative is to place the urethral catheter immediately after surgery.

INTRAOPERATIVE PRECAUTIONS
Skin and Fascial Incision

The direction of the skin incision is likely inconsequential. In 2010, Wylie and colleagues[30] conducted a prospective cohort study and reported quicker infant delivery after a vertical skin incision during emergency cesareans; however, this was not associated with improved neonatal outcomes. Consideration should also be given to the Joel-Cohen entry to effect shorter incision-to-delivery intervals, decreased blood loss, and shorter duration of postoperative pain.[31,32] In 2008, the Cochrane Review reported that Joel-Cohen–based techniques have reductions in operating time, time from skin incision to birth of the infant, blood loss, and fever.[33] The Joel-Cohen entry is achieved with a straight transverse skin incision 3 cm below the level of the anterior superior iliac spines (higher than the Pfannenstiel incision). The subcutaneous layer is opened only in the middle 3 cm. The fascia is incised transversely in the middle and extended laterally with blunt finger dissection. The rectus sheath is separated from the rectus muscles by pulling the sheath caudally and cranially using 2 index fingers.

Uterine Incision

Unless the lower uterine segment is underdeveloped, most surgeons make a low transverse uterine incision. Many obstetricians incise with a scalpel and then extend the incision laterally with their blunt fingers along a path of least resistance. A generous incision is essential to permit optimal room for ease of emergent delivery. Dodd and colleagues[33] discussed 2 trials comparing blunt with sharp dissection to create the transverse hysterotomy. Blunt dissection resulted in a reduction of blood loss. However, Rodriguez and colleagues[34] compared blunt with sharp expansion of low transverse incisions in 286 women at term undergoing nonemergent cesarean births. This randomized prospective study revealed no differences in the incidence of ease of delivery, unintended extension, duration of surgery, estimated blood loss, and postoperative endometritis.[34]

Difficult Fetal Extraction

Challenges may arise in delivery of the fetus through the hysterotomy when the fetal head is either well engaged into the maternal pelvis or high and difficult to descend to the hysterotomy. A vacuum or forceps (eg, Laufe, Barton) and an extra assistant (such as the RN Circulator) should be readily available. With an extra assistant, consideration of application of a vacuum or forceps may aid in delivery. Attempting to deliver an impacted fetal head may cause trauma to the lower uterine segment, vagina, bladder, or ureter. Consideration should be given to the combination of a reverse breech extraction (the pull technique) and assistance from a vaginal hand (the push technique) to facilitate delivery. A reverse breech extraction is achieved as the surgeon introduces a hand through the hysterotomy toward the upper segment of the uterus and, after grasping the fetal legs, gently pulls the fetus through the hysterotomy. During the push technique, the fetal head is dislodged by pushing it through the vagina and the fetus is delivered by routine cesarean delivery. Bastani and colleagues[35] reported a decrease in infection with the pull method and likewise, Veisi and colleagues[36] noted lower maternal morbidity with the pull method.

POSTOPERATIVE PRECAUTIONS
Checklist

Open communication is essential throughout the operative experience. Checklists for open discussion were first introduced in aviation in the 1930s to address human error with the use of increasingly complex aircraft.[37] Likewise, to decrease morbidity and mortality, the World Health Organization designed the Surgical Safety Checklist in 2008 to decrease morbidity and mortality.[38] Levy and colleagues[39] highlighted the importance of staff education and familiarity with checklists and their proper execution. Concern about heightened patient fears with the use of checklists (because patients can be awake) was allayed by Kerans and colleagues[40] who reported lower levels of anxiety and increased patient comfort with the addition of safety checks. Additional concerns about implementing a checklist at the time of an emergent surgery have been alleviated after finding that checklists are equally applicable and may improve the focus of the surgical team.[41,42] Communication and patient outcomes may also be improved with implementation of postoperative debriefings between the obstetrician, anesthesia team, and operating room staff.[38] Listed in **Box 2** is our proposed checklist for emergency cesarean delivery.

Box 2
Emergency cesarean delivery checklist

- Obtain informed consent
- Inform delivery team, anesthesia, and other nursing and pediatric staff; request assistance
- Administer preoperative antibiotics, antacids
- Disconnect pumps and monitors to transfer to the operating room
- Prepare the operating room
- Consider Foley catheter placement, sequential compression devices
- Place Bovie pad
- Prep and drape the patient
- Perform the time-out
- Induction of general anesthesia (if no prior regional anesthesia)
- Proceed with cesarean delivery
- Debrief after surgery
- Maternal continuity of care and follow-up

Conditions for Intensive Care Admission

Women delivered by emergency surgery are more likely to be admitted to the intensive care unit, (ICU).[43] The 2 most common causes of ICU admission are hypertensive disorders of pregnancy and obstetric hemorrhage.[43,44] Other reasons for ICU admission include suspected sepsis, anesthetic complications, pulmonary embolism, amniotic fluid embolism, pulmonary edema, acute fatty liver of pregnancy, abnormal adherence of the placenta, and peripartum cardiomyopathy. These patients greatly benefit from close monitoring, hemodynamic support, nutritional support, and multidisciplinary care.

Less Immediate Postpartum Considerations

The unplanned nature of emergency cesarean delivery challenges the patient to adjust psychologically to her surgery. Waldenstrom and colleagues[45] in 2004 found that 23% of women report a negative birth experience following emergent cesarean delivery, with emotions including fear and disappointment. Postpartum care, including assessment for posttraumatic stress symptoms, is critical for patients after emergent cesarean delivery. Between 24% and 34% of women develop childbirth-related posttraumatic stress symptoms (sleep disorders, flashbacks, anxiety, and fatigue), and this is increased with emergency cesarean deliveries.[46–48] Tham and colleagues[49] found that staff and family members are important to the support for patients undergoing emergency cesarean delivery through the postpartum period. Likewise, emergency cesarean delivery can be associated with unfavorable neonatal outcome, and new mothers may benefit from social work or hospital chaplain consultation. It is prudent to recommend an increased time interval between pregnancies to decrease the risk of uterine rupture in subsequent pregnancies.[50–52] The National Institutes of Health cite an interval of 18 months or less as potentially increasing the risk of uterine rupture.[53]

Simulation Training

Simulation training can improve logistical readiness in emergency situations by increasing familiarity and by practicing communication and teamwork. Such drills are recommended by the Joint Commission and ACOG.[54,55] Lipman and colleagues[56] emphasized the effectiveness of simulation to identify and correct institution-specific obstacles that increase the decision-to-delivery interval during cesarean delivery. This prospective study simulated uterine rupture at the time of trial of labor after a prior cesarean delivery. In this series of emergency cesarean drills, surgical teams were timed according to duration of transport from the labor room to the nearby operating room. They were able to identify institution-specific barriers that delayed transport, such as intravenous line entanglement and transferring the patient to a gurney versus directly to the labor bed.

SUMMARY

To decrease the additional morbidity and mortality associated with emergency cesarean delivery, efforts should be made to periodically educate health care providers on conditions, guidelines, and practices before undertaking immediate surgery. Details described in this article regarding preoperative preparation, time-out protocols, anesthesia, antibiotics, and surgical checklists encourage open communication between team members. Periodic simulation drills are valuable to improve teamwork readiness and enhance communication skills. Close follow-up of patients in the postpartum period is important for immediate intensive care or later for emotional support, evaluation of posttraumatic stress symptoms, and planning of any future pregnancies.

REFERENCES

1. Thomas J, Paranjothy S, James D. National cross sectional survey to determine whether the decision to delivery interval is critical in emergency cesarean section. BMJ 2004;328:1–5.
2. Births: national vital statistics reports. vol. 60, 1, November 3, 2011. Available at: http://www.cdc.gov/nchs/data/nvsr/nvsr60/nvsr60_01.pdf. Accessed August 12, 2012.
3. Bergholt T, Lim LK, Jorgensen JS, et al. Maternal body mass index in the first trimester and risk of cesarean delivery in nulliparous women in spontaneous labor. Am J Obstet Gynecol 2007;196:163–5.
4. Haerskjold A, Hegaard HK, Kjaergaard H. Emergency caesarean section in low risk nulliparous women. J Obstet Gynaecol 2012;32:543–7.
5. American College of Obstetricians and Gynecologists. Optimal goals for anesthesia care in obstetrics. ACOG Committee Opinion #256. Washington, DC: American College of Obstetricians and Gynecologists; 2001.
6. Chauhan SP, Roach H, Naef RW, et al. Cesarean section for suspected fetal distress: does the decision-incision time make a difference? J Reprod Med 1997;42(6):347–52.
7. MacKenzie IZ, Cooke I. What is a reasonable time from decision-to-delivery by cesarean section? Evidence from 415 deliveries. BJOG 2002;109:498.
8. Spencer MK, MacLennan AH. How long does it take to deliver a baby by emergency cesarean section? Aust N Z J Obstet Gynaecol 2001;41:7–11.
9. Cerbinskaite A, Malone S, McDermott J, et al. Emergency caesarean section: influences on the decision-to-delivery interval. J Pregnancy 2011;13:1–6.
10. Leung TY, Chung PW, Rogers MS, et al. Urgent cesarean delivery for fetal bradycardia. Obstet Gynecol 2009;114:1023–8.
11. Smill F, Hofmeyr GJ. Antibiotic prophylaxis for cesarean section. Cochrane Database Syst Rev 2002;(3):CD000933.
12. Dhar H, Dhar D. Informed consent in clinical practice and literature overview. Arch Gynecol Obstet 2012;286:649–51.
13. Berg JW, Appelbaum PS, Lidz CW, et al. Informed consent: legal theory and clinical practice. New York: Oxford University Press; 2001. p. 41–73.
14. Jeejeebhoy FM, Zelop CM, Windrim R, et al. Management of cardiac arrest in pregnancy: a systematic review. Resuscitation 2011;82:801–9.
15. Jones R, Baird S, Thurman S, et al. Maternal cardiac arrest. J Perinat Neonatal Nurs 2012;26:117–23.
16. Committee opinion no. 456. Antimicrobial prophylaxis for cesarean delivery: timing of administration. Obstet Gynecol 2010;116:791–2.
17. Lee CE, Zembower TR, Fotis MA, et al. The incidence of antimicrobial allergies in hospitalized patients: implications regarding prescribing patterns and emerging bacterial resistance. Arch Intern Med 2000;160:2819–22.
18. American College of Obstetricians and Gynecologists. Use of prophylactic antibiotics in labor and delivery. Practice bulletin no. 120. Obstet Gynecol 2011; 117:1472–83.
19. Blanca M, Torres MJ, Garcia JJ, et al. Natural evolution of skin test sensitivity in patients allergic to beta-lactam antibiotics. J Allergy Clin Immunol 1999;103: 918–24.

20. Honiden S, Abdel-Razeq SS, Siegel MD. The management of the critically ill obstetric patient. J Intensive Care Med 2011;8:1–14.
21. American College of Obstetricians and Gynecologists. Obesity in pregnancy. ACOG committee opinion no. 315. Obstet Gynecol 2005;106:671–5.
22. Davies GA, Maxwell C, McLeod L, et al. Obesity in pregnancy. Int J Gynaecol Obstet 2010;110:167–73.
23. Facts about universal protocol. The Joint Commission. Available at: http://www.jointcommission.org/assets/1/6/NPSG_Chapter_Jan2012_HAP.pdf. Accessed September 2, 2012.
24. Conley DM, Singer SJ, Edmondson L, et al. Effective surgical safety checklist implementation. J Am Coll Surg 2011;212:873–9.
25. Vasdev GM, Harrison BA, Keegan MT, et al. Management of the difficult and failed airway in obstetric anesthesia. J Anesth 2008;22:38–48.
26. Popham P, Buettner A, Mendola M. Anaesthesia for emergency caesarean section, 2000-2004, at the Royal Women's Hospital Melbourne. Anaesth Intensive Care 2007;35:74–9.
27. Birnbach DJ, Browne IM. Anesthesia for obstetrics. Miller's Anesthesia 2009;69:2203–40.
28. Li L, Wen J, Wang L, et al. Is routine indwelling catheterization of the bladder for caesarean section necessary? A systematic review. BJOG 2011;118:400–9.
29. Senanayake H. Elective cesarean section without urethral catheterization. J Obstet Gynaecol Res 2005;21:32–7.
30. Wylie BJ, Gilbert S, Landon MB, et al. Comparison of transverse and vertical skin incision for emergency cesarean delivery. Obstet Gynecol 2010;115:1134–40.
31. Mathai M, Hofmeyr GJ. Abdominal surgical incisions for caesarean section. Cochrane Database Syst Rev 2007;(1):CD004453.
32. Hofmeyr GJ, Mathai M, Shah A, et al. Techniques for cesarean section. Cochrane Database Syst Rev 2008;(1):CD004662. http://dx.doi.org/10.1002/14651858.CD004662.pub2.
33. Dodd JM, Anderson ER, Gates S. Surgical techniques for uterine incision and uterine closure at the time of caesarean section. Cochrane Database Syst Rev 2008;(3):CD004732. http://dx.doi.org/10.1002/14651858.CD004732.pub2.
34. Rodriguez AL, Porter KB, O'Brien WR. Blunt versus sharp expansion of the uterine incision in low-segment cesarean section. Am J Obstet Gynecol 1994;171:1022–5.
35. Bastani P, Pourabolghase S, Abbasalizadeh F, et al. Comparison of neonatal and maternal outcomes associated with head-pushing and head-pulling methods for impacted fetal head extraction during cesarean delivery. Int J Gynaecol Obstet 2012;118:1–3.
36. Veisi F, Zangeneh M, Malekkhosravi S, et al. Comparison of "push" and "pull" methods for impacted fetal head extraction during cesarean delivery. Int J Gynaecol Obstet 2012;118:4–6.
37. Weiser T, Haynes A, Lashoher A, et al. Perspectives in quality: designing the WHO Surgical Safety Checklist. Int J Qual Health Care 2010;22:365–70.
38. Haynes AB, Weiser TG, Berry WR, et al. A surgical safety checklist to reduce morbidity and mortality in a global population. N Engl J Med 2009;360:491–9.
39. Levy SM, Senter CE, Hawkins RB, et al. Implementing a surgical checklist: more than checking a box. Surgery 2012;152:331–6.
40. Kerans RJ, Uppal V, Bonner J, et al. The introduction of a surgical checklist in a tertiary referral obstetric centre. BMJ Qual Saf 2011;20:818–20.

41. Weiser T, Haynes A, Dziekan G, et al. Effect of a 19-item surgical safety checklist during urgent operations in a global patient population. Ann Surg 2010;251: 976–80.
42. Hunter DN, Finney SJ. Follow surgical checklists and take time out, especially in a crisis. BMJ 2011;344:d8194.
43. Selo-Ojeme DO, Omosaiye M, Battacharjee P, et al. Risk factors for obstetric admissions to the intensive care unit in a tertiary hospital: a case-control study. Arch Gynecol Obstet 2005;272:201–10.
44. Pollock W, Rose L, Dennis C. Pregnant and postpartum admissions to the intensive care unit: a systematic review. Intensive Care Med 2010;36:1465–74.
45. Waldenström U, Hildingsson I, Rubersson C, et al. A negative birth experience: prevalence and risk factors in a national sample. Birth 2004 Mar;31(1):17–27.
46. Soet J, Brack G, Dilorio C. Prevalence and predictors of women's experience of psychological trauma during childbirth. Birth 2003;30:36–46.
47. Czarnocka J, Slade P. Prevalence and predictors of post-traumatic stress symptoms following childbirth. Br J Clin Psychol 2000;39:35–51.
48. Ayers S. Delivery as a traumatic event: prevalence, risk factors, and treatment for postnatal posttraumatic stress disorder. Clin Obstet Gynecol 2004;47:552–67.
49. Tham V, Ryding EL, Christensson K. Experience of support among mothers with and without post-traumatic stress symptoms following caesarean section. Sex Reprod Healthc 2010;1:175–80.
50. Shipp TD, Zelop CM, Repke JT, et al. Interdelivery interval and risk of symptomatic uterine rupture. Obstet Gynecol 2001;97:175–7.
51. Bujold E, Mehta SH, Bujold C, et al. Interdelivery interval and uterine rupture. Am J Obstet Gynecol 2002;187:1199–202.
52. Esposito MA, Menihan CA, Malee MP. Association of interpregnancy interval with uterine scar failure in labor: a case-control study. Am J Obstet Gynecol 2000;183: 1180–3.
53. Vaginal birth after cesarean: new insights. Obstet Gynecol 2010. Available at: http://consensus.nih.gov/2010/vbacstatement.htm#q1. Accessed September 26, 2012.
54. Preventing infant death and injury during delivery. The Joint Commission 2004. Available at: http://www.jointcommission.org/assets/1/18/SEA_30.PDF. Accessed August 12, 2012.
55. American College of Obstetricians and Gynecologists. Vaginal birth after previous cesarean delivery. Practice bulletin no. 115. Obstet Gynecol 2010;116:450–63.
56. Lipman SS, Carvalho B, Cohen SE, et al. Response times for emergency cesarean delivery: use of simulation drills to assess and improve obstetric team performance. J Perinatol 2012;1–5.

Trauma During Pregnancy

Steffen Brown, MD*, Ellen Mozurkewich, MD, MS

KEYWORDS

- Pregnancy • Trauma • Mortality • Abruption

KEY POINTS

- Trauma is the leading cause of nonobstetric death and affects 6% to 8% of all pregnancies.
- Adverse outcomes of pregnancy, including fetal loss, preterm delivery, and placental abruption, are more frequent following trauma.
- Optimal management includes transport to a site with obstetric services, proper positioning, fetal monitoring, laboratory studies, diagnostic imaging, and in some cases emergency cesarean delivery.

INTRODUCTION

In the United States, traumatic injuries complicate 6% to 8% of pregnancies, causing approximately 30,000 women to seek care for injuries each year.[1–3] The most common causes of trauma in pregnancy include motor vehicle collisions (54.6%), violent assaults (22.3%), and falls (21.8%). Other, less common, causes include suicide attempts, burns, puncture wounds, and animal bites.[4,5]

Several factors portend an increased risk of trauma during pregnancy. These include age less than 20, non-white race, low socioeconomic status, drug use, and alcohol use.[1,6] Intimate partner violence, which affects approximately 324,000 pregnant women per year in the United States, tends to escalate during the pregnancy and postpartum periods.[7]

MATERNAL-FETAL MORTALITY FROM TRAUMA

The leading cause of nonobstetric death in pregnancy is traumatic injury.[8–10] Nonobstetric deaths include those that are not caused by complications of gestation and partuition (direct) or exacerbations of preexisting medical conditions that worsen in pregnancy (indirect). Though other causes of maternal death remain prevalent, traumatic injury is both widespread and burdensome.

Declaration of interest: The authors do not report any potential conflict of interest.
Division of Maternal Fetal Medicine, Department of Obstetrics and Gynecology, University of New Mexico School of Medicine, MSC10 5580, 1 University of New Mexico, Albuquerque, NM 87131, USA
* Corresponding author.
E-mail address: StBrown@salud.unm.edu

Obstet Gynecol Clin N Am 40 (2013) 47–57
http://dx.doi.org/10.1016/j.ogc.2012.11.004
0889-8545/13/$ – see front matter © 2013 Elsevier Inc. All rights reserved.

obgyn.theclinics.com

Trauma during pregnancy leading to maternal or fetal mortality is most often intentional. One Cook County series found 57% of traumatic maternal deaths attributable to homicide and 9% to suicide.[11] A New York City series had similar findings; homicides accounted for 63% and suicides 13%.[12]

The remainder of trauma-associated mortality follows motor vehicle collisions. As is true with the nonpregnant population, pregnant women documented as unrestrained had the highest rates of mortality. The most common cause of death in this setting was head injury.[13–16]

Incidence of fetal mortality is difficult to estimate due to wide variance in mechanisms of reporting. It is clear that fetal loss after maternal trauma does occur as a function of direct trauma, hypotension, placental abruption, and preterm delivery. A review of fetal death certificates in Pennsylvania suggests maternal trauma resulting from motor vehicle collisions causes 90 to 367 deaths of viable fetuses each year in the United States.[17] However, when first and second trimester losses are included, estimates include as many as 4000 fetal deaths per year related to motor vehicle trauma. Although severe trauma commonly leads to fetal loss, minor trauma is so common in pregnancy that these injuries are responsible for 60% to 70% of fetal losses.[3]

ANATOMIC AND PHYSIOLOGIC CHANGES OF PREGNANCY
Maternal Adaptation

The physiologic maternal and fetal response to trauma may influence the severity of trauma as well as the optimal strategy for treatment. An understanding of the fundamental anatomic and physiologic differences that exist in the pregnant state facilitates the proper evaluation and treatment of the maternal response to stress, hypovolemia, and fetal perfusion.

Maternal adaptation to pregnancy involves several organ systems and, in many cases, represents a dramatic departure from the nonpregnant state. The most clinically relevant physiologic changes of pregnancy relate to the evaluation of occult hemorrhage and management of hypotension, including

- Decrease in mean blood pressure of 10 to 15 mm Hg by the second trimester
- Increase in pulse of 5 to 15 beats per minute by the second trimester
- Decrease in hemoglobin to 9 to 11 g/dL due to volume expansion and iron deficiency
- Blood volume increases to approximately 6 L.[18,19]

Management of the airway also carries additional risks in pregnancy. Changes in oncotic pressure and increases in blood volume create an edematous airway, which can lead to difficult intubation. Aspiration risk is increased by the progesterone-mediated delay in gastric emptying and estrogen-mediated relaxation of the esophageal sphincter. Eating patterns in pregnancy, spurred on by common advice to eat frequent, small meals, also increase the likelihood that a pregnant patient presenting with trauma will have a full stomach.

Important anatomic changes of pregnancy are primarily the function of the gravid uterus. Clinically relevant changes include

- Superior displacement of the bowel, with potential for complex and multiple intestinal injuries with penetrating trauma of the upper abdomen
- Hypertrophied pelvic vasculature, with potential for massive retroperitoneal hemorrhage in the event of pelvic fracture
- Uterine compression of the inferior vena cava, with potential for impairment of up to 00% of cardiac output during supine positioning.[19]

Fetal Structure and Function

Fetal anatomic and physiologic changes relevant to trauma in pregnancy include factors that predispose to maternal exsanguination and placental abruption and alter the process of maternal resuscitation. First, the growing fetus draws uterine blood flow of up to 600 mL per minute.[19] In the event of laceration of the uterine vasculature or rupture of the uterus, rapid maternal exsanguination can occur unless emergent delivery and repair are achieved.

Second, the growing placental mass creates a large, relatively inelastic, vascular conduit capable of facilitating rapid maternal and fetal exsanguination in the case of abruption.[20] Finally, the algorithm for resuscitation of the perimortem pregnant patient allows for consideration of fetal perfusion after the age of viability, a center-specific gestational age after which the fetus has the potential to independently survive.[21] These fetal changes create several areas of vulnerability to poor outcomes in the event of trauma.

PREDICTING OUTCOME AFTER TRAUMA
Maternal Outcomes

Short-term and intermediate outcomes for pregnant trauma victims may be worse than nonpregnant controls, even for minor injuries.[22] Conversely, mortality among pregnant trauma victims is likely lower than nonpregnant controls.[13] As with the nonpregnant patient, injury severity score predicts maternal outcome. Maternal abdominal injuries may produce worse outcomes than other score-matched injuries.[23]

Fetal Outcomes

Prediction of fetal outcomes after trauma depends on the mechanism and severity of injury. Fetal loss is frequent after penetrating trauma to the uterus, including gunshot wounds (71%) and stabbings (42%).[24] Placental abruption is the leading cause of fetal death after trauma, accounting for 50% to 70% of all trauma-related fetal losses. Rates of placental abruption vary by mechanism and tend to be highest with severe motor vehicle collisions (50%), maternal assaults (5%), and falls (3%).[17,25,26] After abruption, maternal death is the second most frequent cause of trauma-associated fetal deaths; an estimated 10% of trauma-related fetal losses follow maternal death.[25]

Schiff and Holt[27] used injury severity score to assess the risk of fetal loss after maternal injury. Although the most severe maternal injuries were most likely to lead to adverse obstetric outcome, the severity score had otherwise limited negative predictive value for fetal outcome. By contrast, the extent to which minor injuries such as falls pose risk for adverse fetal outcomes is controversial.[17] For example, in a series of 317 pregnant women with minor trauma, evaluation of the variables: positive Kleihauer-Betke (KB) test, fibrinogen less than 200, more than 5 contractions per hour, abdominal pain, anterior placenta, and direct abdominal trauma found that none of them were predictive of composite adverse outcome.[28] In this series, there was only one placental abruption diagnosed many weeks after the traumatic event, suggesting that risk for adverse pregnancy outcomes after minor trauma is low.[28] By contrast, other investigators have reported that even minor maternal injuries may result in fetal loss.[29] A recent retrospective review identified an injury severity score greater than 2 in the presence of a positive KB test as an effective predictor of patients at risk for adverse perinatal outcomes.[30] It seems that risk is increased for both short-term and long-term adverse perinatal outcomes, particularly with more severe trauma.[31]

Minor trauma has also been associated with other adverse outcomes, including preterm labor and delivery, fetal distress, fetal hypoxia, cesarean delivery, and postnatal development of childhood attention-deficit hyperactivity disorder.[29,32] A review of 78,176 deliveries in Tennessee found a correlation between minor injuries during the first and second trimester and subsequent fetal demise, preterm delivery, and low birth weight.[33]

EVALUATION AND MANAGEMENT OF TRAUMA IN PREGNANCY

Care for injuries sustained during trauma in pregnancy often begins with first responders. In the field and in the emergency department, identification of injuries and stabilization of the mother is the clear first priority. In most cases, maternal resuscitation is the safest, fastest means of initial fetal resuscitation. Guidelines for emergency personnel providing care include

- Position in the left lateral decubitus position to relieve compression of the inferior vena cava
- During initial evaluation, leftward tilt of the spinal immobilization board can be achieved with a 6-inch rolled towel[21]
- If possible, transport all pregnancies beyond 20 weeks to a trauma center with obstetric services.[34,35]

Ideal care for the injured pregnant patient includes a multidisciplinary team of emergency medicine providers, trauma surgeons, and obstetricians. The authors suggest that in the viable fetus (beyond 23–24 weeks) a brief initial assessment of fetal heart rate and well-being should be performed in the emergency department. However, fetal assessment should not deter from the initial efforts of maternal resuscitation; delays in correction of maternal hypovolemia and hypoxia are counterproductive to care for the fetus. Once clearance for life-threatening maternal injury is achieved in the emergency department, viable pregnancies should begin extended observation in the labor and delivery suite.

Assessment of Fetal Well-being

Because even minor injuries may be associated with placental abruption and other adverse obstetric outcomes, fetal monitoring after trauma is recommended.[33] Clinical correlates of placental abruption include abdominal pain, vaginal bleeding, and in almost every case, uterine contractions.[36] Although many placental abruptions may be detected by ultrasound, the sensitivity of ultrasound to detect abruption is about 40% in the trauma setting.[37] Because preterm labor following trauma is also a concern, fetal heart rate tracing and tocometry remain the surveillance modality of choice.

Fetal middle cerebral arterial Doppler studies may have a role in fetal assessment after maternal trauma in some cases. In severe cases of fetal anemia following placental abruption and/or maternofetal hemorrhage, the peak systolic velocity of the fetal middle cerebral artery demonstrates a characteristic increase reflective of fetal brain sparing. Ultrasound measurement of this parameter may aid in the identification of fetal hemorrhage in otherwise ambiguous cases.[25,38] The academic or hypoxemic fetus will display a progressive loss of normal fetal behavior. Thus, a biophysical profile may at times be a helpful adjunct to the fetal heart tracing and tocometer.

The presence or absence of uterine contractions may also be helpful in assessing the risk of placental abruption after minor trauma. Placental abruption is unlikely to occur in patients with contractions less frequent than every 15 minutes for more than 4 hours of observation.[39,40] Patients without contractions for more than 4 hours of monitoring following minor trauma may be appropriate for discharge. However, the presence of contractions, other clinical or laboratory signs of placental abruption, a history of direct abdominal trauma, or fetal distress should lead to extended monitoring. Placental abruption can present up to 48 hours after trauma; a minimum of 24 hours of fetal surveillance is recommended for the viable fetus with a high-risk presentation.[25,41]

Laboratory Evaluation

Laboratory testing is directed toward identification of trauma sequelae, including acute blood loss anemia, disseminated intravascular coagulopathy, and maternofetal hemorrhage. As such, the low-risk, Rh-positive patient who has sustained minor trauma, may only require screening for illicit drugs and alcohol. The possible exception to this principle is the use of the KB test, an acid elution quantification of fetal blood in the maternal circulation, to assess risk for adverse perinatal outcome. The KB has been suggested as a means of triaging patients into a higher risk group for preterm delivery and, more recently, multiple adverse perinatal outcomes.[30,42] These uses remain experimental, but should lend caution when considering early discharge.

The KB is potentially useful in the Rh-negative patient; fetomaternal hemorrhage is four times more common in trauma-exposed pregnancies when compared with controls.[43] Although empiric intramuscular Rho(D) immune globulin in the Rh-negative patient is likely to prevent sensitization in most cases, approximately 10% of traumas lead to a fetomaternal hemorrhage exceeding the coverage of a single vial of intramuscular Rho(D) immune globulin (30 mL).[41] Identification of this population for administration of additional intramuscular Rho(D) immune globulin should prevent future adverse perinatal outcomes related to Rh sensitization.

In patients with a fetomaternal hemorrhage greater than 30mL of fetal blood, additional Rho(D) immune globulin should be given as follows: multiply the percentage of fetal cells by 50 to estimate the volume of hemorrhage and give at least an additional 300mcg Rho(D) immune globulin per 15mL of hemorrhage. Individual blood banks often round up or add an additional vial of Rho(D) immune globulin in order to avoid underdosage.[44]

In the setting of severe trauma, internal bleeding, or placental abruption, it is reasonable to perform evaluation of the complete blood count, prothrombin time, partial thromboplastin time, and fibrinogen. Urinalysis may reveal hematuria in the setting of urinary tract injury.[24] Given the strong association between trauma in pregnancy and drug and alcohol abuse, urine toxicology screening is also recommended. Fetal fibronectin has not been evaluated for the prediction of preterm delivery after trauma, though it has proved to predict preterm delivery in other settings.[45]

Diagnostic Imaging

Ionizing radiation

In the setting of severe maternal trauma, future theoretical risks to the fetus should be weighed against the risk to the fetus and mother of undiagnosed maternal injury. Indicated diagnostic procedures to evaluate life or limb-threatening injuries, considered standard of care in the nonpregnant patient, should not be delayed or abandoned due to concerns about fetal radiation.[46,47]

Teratogenesis and carcinogenesis are the main theoretical concerns after in utero ionizing radiation exposure. The levels of ionizing radiation required to cause microcephaly or mental retardation far exceed the doses incurred in common clinical use (**Table 1**). In utero exposure to a 50 mGy (5 rad) dose of ionizing radiation may be associated with a 2% lifetime attributable risk of malignancy. This dose still allows for most common radiologic procedure to be safely performed, including a single-phase CT scan of the abdomen and pelvis (**Table 2**).[48]

Table 1
Effects of in utero exposure to ionizing radiation

Menstrual	<50 mGy (<5 rad)	50–100 mGy (5–10 rad)	>100 mGy (>10 rad)
>27 wk	None	None	None at diagnostic doses
18th and 27th wk	None	None	IQ deficits not detectable at diagnostic doses
11th and 17th wk	None	Potential effects are uncertain and likely minimal	Increased risk of deficits in IQ or mental retardation that increase in frequency and severity with increasing dose.
5th and 10th wk	None	Potential effects are uncertain and likely minimal	Possible malformations increasing in likelihood as dose increases.
3rd and 4th wk	None	Likely none	Possible spontaneous abortion.
0–2 wk	None	None	None

Data from American College of Radiology. ACR practice guideline for imaging pregnant or potentially pregnant adolescents and women with ionizing radiation. Reston (VA): American College of Radiology, 2008.

It is preferable to perform a single CT scan with iodinated contrast rather than perform multiple suboptimal studies without contrast.[48] Although iodinated contrast agents cross the placenta and may be taken up by the fetal thyroid, no cases of fetal goiter or abnormal neonatal thyroid function have been reported in connection with in utero contrast exposure.[49]

With the exception of low-risk, nonpenetrating abdominal injury, most diagnostic imaging of the pregnant trauma victim begins with an obstetric ultrasound and a study requiring the use of ionizing radiation (**Fig. 1**).

MRI

The use of MRI may be a helpful modality in pregnancy because there are no known associated adverse fetal outcomes related to it use. Although the Food and Drug Administration considers the safety of MRI to not be established, there are no reports of adverse perinatal outcomes or long-term pediatric outcomes related to MRI use in pregnancy.[46–48] Currently the use of gadolinium in pregnancy is controversial. In rare instances, gadolinium exposure has resulted in a syndrome of nephrogenic systemic

Table 2
Radiation doses of common diagnostic procedures for traumatic injury

Procedure	Fetal Dose (mGy)
Fluoroscopy of abdomen and pelvis	<100
Single-phase CT scan of abdomen, pelvis, and lumbar spine	<35
CT scan chest view	<1
CT scan head	<1
Hip film (single view)	200 mrad
Chest radiograph	0.02–0.07 mrad

Data from ACOG Committee Opinion #299. Guidelines for diagnostic imaging during pregnancy. Obstet Gynecol 2004;104:647–51; and American College of Radiology. ACR practice guideline for imaging pregnant or potentially pregnant adolescents and women with ionizing radiation. Reston (VA): American College of Radiology, 2008.

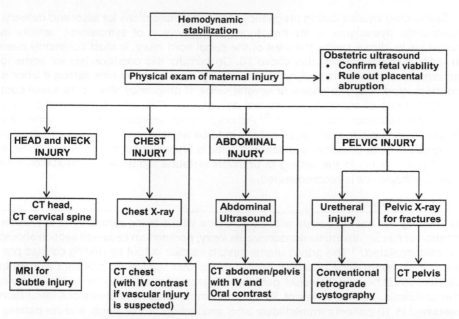

Fig. 1. Algorithm for diagnostic imaging studies for pregnant trauma victims. (*Modified from* Patel SJ, Reede DL, Katz DS, et al. Imaging the pregnant patient for nonobstetric conditions: algorithms and radiation dose considerations. Radiographics 2007;27:1719; with permission.)

fibrosis in children and adults with renal insufficiency. Thus, it is recommended that use of this agent be avoided during pregnancy except when absolutely necessary for adequate imaging.[48] The most vexing problem for use of MRI in evaluation of trauma in pregnancy may be the absence of a well-defined role in management of life-threatening traumatic injuries.

Ultrasound

Abdominal ultrasound is a rapid and safe way to evaluate the pregnant trauma victim for fetal well-being and intraperitoneal hemorrhage. Safety of the use of real-time gray-scale ultrasound in pregnancy is well-established, though concerns remain regarding the mechanical and heat-related effects of prolonged Doppler interrogation.[50] In addition to the parameters of fetal well-being discussed previously, the most relevant use of ultrasound for trauma patients is assessment of free intraperitoneal fluid. Although sensitivity for intraperitoneal hemorrhage is limited to 61% to 83%, specificity has been reported from 94% to 100%.[46]

SPECIAL CONSIDERATIONS
Route of Delivery

Following successful resuscitation and treatment after trauma, the laboring process seems daunting to many patients and providers. However, there are very few injuries that necessitate cesarean delivery. Pelvic fractures have been suggested as a contra-indication to vaginal delivery when the fracture obstructs the birth canal or is unstable. One series found that greater than 80% of women who sustained pelvic fractures could deliver vaginally.[51] An associated bladder or urethral injury may also be a concern.[1]

Spinal cord injuries during pregnancy also carry implications for labor and delivery. Autonomic dysreflexia, a life-threatening exaggeration of sympathetic activity in response to stimuli below the level of the spinal cord injury, is most commonly seen in labor in spinal cord injuries above T6. Concern for this condition has led some to recommend invasive hemodynamic monitoring in an intensive care setting if labor is contemplated.[52] In one review of several series of pregnancy after acute spinal cord injury, the rate of spontaneous vaginal delivery was 37%, operative vaginal delivery 31%, and cesarean delivery 32%.[53] Although newer series also reflect a higher rate of cesarean section, there does not seem to be an increased incidence of failure to progress or fetal intolerance of labor.[54] Little is known about the risks and benefits of vaginal delivery in the setting of unstable vertebral injuries and consultation with spinal orthopedics is recommended.

Perimortem Cesarean

In the pregnant trauma patient with a viable fetus who is failing cardiopulmonary resuscitation or has an obviously nonsurvivable injury, perimortem cesarean section should be contemplated.[21] The gravid uterus inhibits cardiac output by limiting cardiac preload. Early emergency cesarean seems to improve survival for pregnant women in cardiac arrest beyond 20 weeks gestational age or whose the uterine fundus is above the umbilicus. In one series of 20 perimortem cesareans, spontaneous circulation resumed in 12 patients immediately after evacuation of the uterus and no patients experienced a worsening in status.[55]

Perinatal outcomes are optimized when delivery is performed within 5 minutes of cessation of maternal circulation.[35] Beyond 30 minutes, benefit has not been demonstrated.[21] The American Heart Association and others have recommended, and the authors agree, that cesarean delivery should be initiated within 4 minutes after maternal cardiac arrest if resuscitation has failed to restore circulation.[21,25]

SUMMARY

Trauma in pregnancy is a common and morbid event. The most common causes of trauma in pregnancy include motor vehicle collisions, assault, and fall. Even minor trauma can lead to adverse perinatal outcomes such as preterm birth, low birth weight, placental abruption, and fetal loss. Challenges to the obstetrician include adjusting resuscitation strategies to the gravid state, conducting urgent fetal evaluation in the emergency setting, coordinating a multidisciplinary team, advocating for indicated diagnostic imaging, and monitoring for placental abruption and other adverse outcomes.

REFERENCES

1. Mirza FG, Devine PC, Gaddipati S. Trauma in pregnancy: a systematic approach. Am J Perinatol 2010;27(7):579–86.
2. Pearlman MD. Motor vehicle crashes, pregnancy loss and preterm labor. Int J Gynaecol Obstet 1997;57(2):127–32.
3. El Kady D. Perinatal outcomes of traumatic injuries during pregnancy. Clin Obstet Gynecol 2007;50(3):582–91.
4. Connolly AM, Katz VL, Bash KL, et al. Trauma and pregnancy. Am J Perinatol 1997;14(6):331–6.
5. El-Kady D, Gilbert WM, Anderson J, et al. Trauma during pregnancy: an analysis of maternal and fetal outcomes in a large population. Am J Obstet Gynecol 2004; 190(6):1661–8.
6. Oxford CM, Ludmir J. Trauma in pregnancy. Clin Obstet Gynecol 2009;52(4):611–29.

7. ACOG committee opinion no. 518: intimate partner violence. Obstet Gynecol 2012;119(2 Pt 1):412–7.
8. Romero VC, Pearlman M. Maternal mortality due to trauma. Semin Perinatol 2012; 36(1):60–7.
9. Callaghan WM. Overview of maternal mortality in the United States. Semin Perinatol 2012;36(1):2–6.
10. Minino AM, Murphy SL, Xu J, et al. Deaths: final data for 2008. Natl Vital Stat Rep 2011;59(10):1–126.
11. Fildes J, Reed L, Jones N, et al. Trauma: the leading cause of maternal death. J Trauma 1992;32(5):643–5.
12. Dannenberg AL, Carter DM, Lawson HW, et al. Homicide and other injuries as causes of maternal death in New York City, 1987 through 1991. Am J Obstet Gynecol 1995;172(5):1557–64.
13. John PR, Shiozawa A, Haut ER, et al. An assessment of the impact of pregnancy on trauma mortality. Surgery 2011;149(1):94–8.
14. Schiff M, Albers L, McFeeley P. Motor vehicle crashes and maternal mortality in New Mexico: the significance of seat belt use. West J Med 1997;167(1):19–22.
15. Shah KH, Simons RK, Holbrook T, et al. Trauma in pregnancy: maternal and fetal outcomes. J Trauma 1998;45(1):83–6.
16. Crosby WM, Costiloe JP. Safety of lap-belt restraint for pregnant victims of automobile collisions. N Engl J Med 1971;284(12):632–6.
17. Weiss HB, Songer TJ, Fabio A. Fetal deaths related to maternal injury. JAMA 2001;286(15):1863–8.
18. Pearlman M, Faro S. Obstetric septic shock: a pathophysiologic basis for management. Clin Obstet Gynecol 1990;33(3):482–92.
19. Wilkening RB, Meschia G. Fetal oxygen uptake, oxygenation, and acid-base balance as a function of uterine blood flow. Am J Physiol 1983;244(6):H749–55.
20. Pérés J, Thollon L, Delotte J, et al. Material properties of the placenta under dynamic loading conditions. Comput Methods Biomech Biomed Engin 2012. http://dx.doi.org/10.1080/10255842.2012.727403.
21. Vanden Hoek TL, Morrison LJ, Shuster M, et al. Part 12: cardiac arrest in special situations: 2010 American heart association guidelines for cardiopulmonary resuscitation and emergency cardiovascular care. Circulation 2010;122(18 Suppl 3): S829–61.
22. Cheng HT, Wang YC, Lo HC, et al. Trauma during pregnancy: a population-based analysis of maternal outcome. World J Surg 2012;36:2767–75.
23. Petrone P, Talving P, Browder T, et al. Abdominal injuries in pregnancy: a 155-month study at two level 1 trauma centers. Injury 2011;42(1):47–9.
24. Brown HL. Trauma in pregnancy. Obstet Gynecol 2009;114(1):147–60.
25. Muench MV, Canterino JC. Trauma in pregnancy. Obstet Gynecol Clin North Am 2007;34(3):555–83, xiii.
26. El Kady D, Gilbert WM, Xing G, et al. Maternal and neonatal outcomes of assaults during pregnancy. Obstet Gynecol 2005;105(2):357–63.
27. Schiff MA, Holt VL. The injury severity score in pregnant trauma patients: predicting placental abruption and fetal death. J Trauma 2002;53(5):946–9.
28. Cahill AG, Bastek JA, Stamilio DM, et al. Minor trauma in pregnancy—is the evaluation unwarranted? Am J Obstet Gynecol 2008;198(2):208.e1–5.
29. Schiff MA. Pregnancy outcomes following hospitalisation for a fall in Washington State from 1987 to 2004. BJOG 2008;115(13):1648–54.
30. Trivedi N, Ylagan M, Moore TR, et al. Predicting adverse outcomes following trauma in pregnancy. J Reprod Med 2012;57(1–2):3–8.

31. Melamed N, Aviram A, Silver M, et al. Pregnancy course and outcome following blunt trauma. J Matern Fetal Neonatal Med 2012;25(9):1612–7.
32. Amiri S, Malek A, Sadegfard M, et al. Pregnancy-related maternal risk factors of attention-deficit hyperactivity disorder: a case-control study. ISRN Pediatr 2012; 2012:458064.
33. Fischer PE, Zarzaur BL, Fabian TC, et al. Minor trauma is an unrecognized contributor to poor fetal outcomes: a population-based study of 78,552 pregnancies. J Trauma 2011;71(1):90–3.
34. Sasser SM, Hunt RC, Sullivent EE, et al. Guidelines for field triage of injured patients. recommendations of the national expert panel on field triage. MMWR Recomm Rep 2009;58(RR-1):1–35.
35. Tsuei BJ. Assessment of the pregnant trauma patient. Injury 2006;37(5):367–73.
36. Pearlman MD, Tintinallli JE, Lorenz RP. A prospective controlled study of outcome after trauma during pregnancy. Am J Obstet Gynecol 1990;162(6):1502–7 [discussion: 1507–10].
37. Williams JK, McClain L, Rosemurgy AS, et al. Evaluation of blunt abdominal trauma in the third trimester of pregnancy: maternal and fetal considerations. Obstet Gynecol 1990;75(1):33–7.
38. Cosmi E, Rampon M, Saccardi C, et al. Middle cerebral artery peak systolic velocity in the diagnosis of fetomaternal hemorrhage. Int J Gynaecol Obstet 2012;117(2):128–30.
39. Klinich KD, Flannagan CA, Rupp JD, et al. Fetal outcome in motor-vehicle crashes: effects of crash characteristics and maternal restraint. Am J Obstet Gynecol 2008;198(4):450.e1–9.
40. Dahmus MA, Sibai BM. Blunt abdominal trauma: are there any predictive factors for abruptio placentae or maternal-fetal distress? Am J Obstet Gynecol 1993; 169(4):1054–9.
41. Williams J, Mozurkewich E, Chilimigras J, et al. Critical care in obstetrics: pregnancy-specific conditions. Best Pract Res Clin Obstet Gynaecol 2008; 22(5):825–46.
42. Muench MV, Baschat AA, Reddy UM, et al. Kleihauer-betke testing is important in all cases of maternal trauma. J Trauma 2004;57(5):1094–8.
43. Chames MC, Pearlman MD. Trauma during pregnancy: outcomes and clinical management. Clin Obstet Gynecol 2008;51(2):398–408.
44. Moise K. Hemolytic disease of the fetus and newborn. In: Creasy and Resnik's maternal-fetal medicine: principles and practice. 6th edition. Philadelphia: Saunders Elsevier; 2009. p. 480–1.
45. Sanchez-Ramos L, Delke I, Zamora J, et al. Fetal fibronectin as a short-term predictor of preterm birth in symptomatic patients: a meta-analysis. Obstet Gynecol 2009;114(3):631–40.
46. Patel SJ, Reede DL, Katz DS, et al. Imaging the pregnant patient for nonobstetric conditions: algorithms and radiation dose considerations. Radiographics 2007; 27(6):1705–22.
47. Puri A, Khadem P, Ahmed S, et al. Imaging of trauma in a pregnant patient. Semin Ultrasound CT MR 2012;33(1):37–45.
48. Chen MM, Coakley FV, Kaimal A, et al. Guidelines for computed tomography and magnetic resonance imaging use during pregnancy and lactation. Obstet Gynecol 2008;112(2 Pt 1):333–40.
49. Lee I, Chew FS. Use of IV iodinated and gadolinium contrast media in the pregnant or lactating patient: self-assessment module. AJR Am J Roentgenol 2009; 100(Quppl 0):070 0.

50. Sheiner E, Abramowicz JS. A symposium on obstetrical ultrasound: is all this safe for the fetus? Clin Obstet Gynecol 2012;55(1):188–98.
51. Gunter J, Pearlman M. Emergencies during pregnancy: trauma and nonobstetric surgical conditions. In: Ling F, Duff P, editors. Obstetrics and gynecology: principles for practice. New York: McGraw-Hill; 2001. p. 253.
52. Hughes SJ, Short DJ, Usherwood MM, et al. Management of the pregnant woman with spinal cord injuries. Br J Obstet Gynaecol 1991;98(6):513–8.
53. Pereira L. Obstetric management of the patient with spinal cord injury. Obstet Gynecol Surv 2003;58(10):678–87.
54. Signore C, Spong CY, Krotoski D, et al. Pregnancy in women with physical disabilities. Obstet Gynecol 2011;117(4):935–47.
55. Katz V, Balderston K, DeFreest M. Perimortem cesarean delivery: were our assumptions correct? Am J Obstet Gynecol 2005;192(6):1916–20 [discussion: 1920–1].

Shoulder Dystocia

William Grobman, MD, MBA

KEYWORDS

- Shoulder dystocia • Obstetric emergency • Simulation

KEY POINTS

- Shoulder dystocia is a relatively uncommon and unpredictable obstetric emergency.
- Once a shoulder dystocia is recognized, alleviating maneuvers should be used; however, there is no consensus that a particular sequence of alleviating maneuvers is preferred.
- Simulations have been associated with a reduced frequency of brachial plexus palsies in longitudinal studies; it remains unknown whether such simulations can reduce the probability of longer-lasting brachial plexus palsies.

HOW FREQUENT IS SHOULDER DYSTOCIA?

From a clinical standpoint, a shoulder dystocia is most often diagnosed when the typical gentle downward traction on the fetal head that is used to deliver the anterior shoulder is not sufficient to enact this delivery or when ancillary obstetric maneuvers are required to engender delivery of the fetal shoulders.

As can be surmised from the clinical definition, there is a certain degree of subjectivity related to the diagnosis of shoulder dystocia. Accordingly, the frequency of shoulder dystocia in different reports has varied, ranging from 0.2% to 3% of all vaginal deliveries.[1] To remove the subjective component, some investigators have attempted to establish an objective standard for the diagnosis of shoulder dystocia. One group, for example, assessed whether shoulder dystocia could be defined according to the length of time between delivery of the fetal head and the fetal body. This group could not, however, find a threshold that clearly distinguished deliveries complicated by shoulder dystocia from those without shoulder dystocia.[2] Ultimately, there is no consensus as to whether there is a time threshold or any other objective measure that explicitly indicates that a shoulder dystocia has occurred. Consequently, the diagnosis of shoulder dystocia continues to depend on the clinician who is assisting with the delivery and his or her perception of whether the typical downward traction that is typically used to accomplish delivery of the fetal shoulders is not effective.

Feinberg School of Medicine, Northwestern University, 250 East Superior Street, Suite 05-2175, Chicago, IL 60611, USA
E-mail address: w-grobman@northwestern.edu

Obstet Gynecol Clin N Am 40 (2013) 59–67
http://dx.doi.org/10.1016/j.ogc.2012.11.006
0889-8545/13/$ – see front matter © 2013 Elsevier Inc. All rights reserved.

WHAT ADVERSE OUTCOMES ARE ASSOCIATED WITH SHOULDER DYSTOCIA?

Once a shoulder dystocia occurs, and even if all actions are appropriately taken, there is an increased incidence of both maternal and neonatal trauma. Reported maternal complications related to shoulder dystocia have included third- or fourth-degree perineal lacerations, postpartum hemorrhage, vaginal or cervical lacerations, and symphyseal separation with lateral femoral cutaneous neuropathy. Self-limiting neonatal complications include clavicular and humeral fracture, which occur in approximately 5% to 10% of shoulder dystocia cases.[3] In addition, brachial plexus palsies—predominantly of the Erb-Duchenne (C5 through C6) or the Klumpke (C8 through T1) type—occur in 10% to 20% of neonates born after a shoulder dystocia. Fortunately, most of these neurologic conditions resolve over time, with an estimated rate of persistence of 1% to 5%.[4] Other long-term neonatal complications that have been reported to occur, albeit infrequently, include permanent central neurologic injury and death.[5] However, there is not good evidence that complications such as brachial plexus palsy can be completely prevented even when a shoulder dystocia is managed appropriately. Indeed, brachial plexus palsies have been noted to occur even in the absence of apparent shoulder dystocia. For example, Torki and colleagues[6] reported on 8 cases without shoulder dystocia but with severe brachial plexus palsy requiring neonatal intensive care unit admission. None of the patients had maternal diabetes, previous shoulder dystocia, or previous macrosomia and none of them had undergone labor induction. One, in fact, was delivered by cesarean.

CAN SHOULDER DYSTOCIA BE ACCURATELY PREDICTED?

Multiple risk factors have been reported to be associated with shoulder dystocia, including maternal diabetes mellitus, maternal obesity, prolonged second stage of labor, precipitous second stage of labor, operative vaginal delivery, birth weight, gestational age at delivery, and prior shoulder dystocia. However, many of these reported associations are not independent or have been demonstrated inconsistently.[7] Moreover, even for the factors that have been consistently and independently associated with shoulder dystocia, there has not been good evidence that their use can allow accurate prediction of the condition.[3,8] For example, shoulder dystocia increases in frequency as the birth weight increases. In one study, 5.2% of nondiabetic mothers with neonates who weighed 4000 to 4250 g experienced shoulder dystocia, compared with 21.1% of mothers whose infants weighed 4750 to 5000 g.[9] Nevertheless, approximately 40% to 60% of shoulder dystocias occur in infants weighing less than 4000 g.[3] Dodd and colleagues[10] are one of the most recent in a line of investigators to try and determine whether, using known risk factors, shoulder dystocia could be accurately predicted. Their conclusion, echoing those of prior investigators, is that "(w)hile there are a number of factors associated with an increased risk of shoulder dystocia, none are of sufficient sensitivity or positive predictive value to allow their use clinically to reliably and accurately identify the occurrence of shoulder dystocia."

One risk factor for shoulder dystocia that deserves attention is "history of a shoulder dystocia," because recurrence rates are increased in a subsequent pregnancy, particularly when the fetus is of similar or greater size.[11] In women who have had a shoulder dystocia, the probability of having a recurrence that is further complicated by a birth injury has been noted to be greater with birth weight of 4000 g or more (adjusted odds ratio [aOR], 4.4; 95% confidence interval [CI], 3.0–6.3), gestational diabetes (aOR, 1.9; 95% CI, 1.2–3.2), Hispanic ethnicity (aOR, 1.9; 95% CI, 1.2–2.9), and maternal obesity (aOR 1.8; 95% CI, 1.3–2.6).[12] Yet, the vast majority of parturients do not have the risk factor of a "prior shoulder dystocia," but among the risk factor in addition to those mentioned above. Thus, from a prospective point of view, physicians have a poor ability to predict shoulder dystocia for most patients and there remains no commonly accepted model to accurately predict this obstetric emergency.

Although some have advocated that fetal weight should be estimated by sonography during the late third trimester or the intrapartum period and then be used to estimate the risk and reduce the frequency of shoulder dystocia, such weight estimates are not very sensitive for detecting birth weight thresholds (such as >4000 g or >4500 g).[13] In fact, investigators have found that the accuracy of sonography is no better than that of clinical palpation or of a parous woman's assessment of her own fetus' weight.[14] More importantly, management change based on estimated fetal weight has not been shown to significantly reduce the frequency of shoulder dystocia. For example, some have advocated that women with suspected or impending fetal "macrosomia" undergo labor induction to reduce their risk of cesarean delivery and shoulder dystocia. However, there is no good evidence to support this practice. In one prospective clinical trial, nondiabetic patients with ultrasonographic fetal weight estimation of 4000 to 4500 g who were randomized to induction of labor had a frequency of shoulder dystocia that was no different than that of the women who were randomized to expectant manage-ment.[15] Similarly, cesarean delivery as a prophylactic intervention based on estimated fetal weight has not been demonstrated to significantly reduce shoulder dystocia without incurring significant increases in the frequency of cesarean delivery and its associated complications.[4,16] Nevertheless, expert opinion, based on the epidemio-logic data that do exist, states that it is reasonable to offer prophylactic cesarean delivery for an estimated fetal weight greater than 5000 g in women without diabetes or greater than 4500 g in women with diabetes.[14]

WHAT SHOULD BE DONE WHEN A SHOULDER DYSTOCIA OCCURS?

In some cases, shoulder dystocia may be indicated by the "turtle sign," during which the fetal head, after it has delivered, retracts back tightly against the maternal peri-neum. Under these circumstances, some clinicians have advocated immediately using maneuvers to effect delivery of the fetal shoulders to maintain the forward momentum of the fetus. Others, however, have suggested that it is better to allow a short delay in delivery of the shoulders, given that the endogenous rotational mechanics of the second stage may spontaneously alleviate the obstruction. Data that exist do not allow definitive determination of which is the better approach.

Regardless, once shoulder dystocia is recognized, either by a "turtle" sign or the lack of delivery of the anterior shoulder after typical gentle downward traction on the fetal head, alleviating maneuvers should be used. These maneuvers include some combination of the McRoberts maneuver, suprapubic pressure, fetal rotation, or delivery of the fetal posterior arm. Many providers first turn to McRoberts maneuver or suprapubic pressure (or both) because of the ease of implementation, relatively high success rate (approximately 40%–60%), and involvement of only maternal manipula-tion.[3] McRoberts maneuver describes the exaggerated abduction and hyperflexion of the maternal thighs upon the abdomen. When a woman is placed in this position, the actual dimensions of the maternal pelvis are not changed, but instead, the symphysis pubis is caudally rotated and the sacrum is flattened[17]; these changes in pelvic orien-tation are believed to facilitate delivery. Despite being useful, once a shoulder dystocia has occurred, the McRoberts maneuver and/or suprapubic pressure has not been shown to be helpful as prophylactic measures to try to avoid shoulder dystocia.[18]

Other techniques that may be helpful in resolving shoulder dystocia involve fetal manipulation. One type of technique is the rotational maneuver, in which the operator rotates the fetus to an oblique, rather than the anteroposterior axis, thereby allowing disimpaction of the anterior shoulder from the symphysis pubis. Many different variations of rotational maneuvers have been described; 2 that are commonly referred to are the Wood and Rubin maneuvers. In the former, the practitioner attempts to rotate the fetus by exerting pressure on the anterior surface of the posterior shoulder and pushing toward the fetal back. In the latter, the practitioner applies pressure to the posterior surface of either the posterior or the anterior fetal shoulder and pushes toward the fetal chest, an action that also may assist in the alleviation of the dystocia by causing shoulder adduction. Another type of alleviating action is the delivery of the posterior arm. To perform this maneuver, the provider should apply pressure at the antecubital fossa to flex the fetal forearm and then sweep the arm across the fetus' chest, with ultimate delivery of the arm over the perineum. After delivery of the arm, there is a 20% reduction in shoulder diameter, thereby allowing the dystocia to be relieved.[19]

Although episiotomy may be used in the setting of shoulder dystocia, there is not good evidence that this is a maneuver that should be routinely used or that it results in better clinical outcomes. For example, Paris and colleagues[20] studied all 94,842 deliveries at their institution over 10 years. In the presence of a shoulder dystocia, episiotomy became significantly less frequent over time (40%–4%, $P = .005$) with no change in the rate of brachial plexus palsies. Nevertheless, even if episiotomy is not a mandatory procedure, the operator may decide, given the individual circumstances, that an episiotomy will allow other maneuvers to be accomplished more easily or effectively, in which case an episiotomy is an acceptable choice. On the other hand, one maneuver for which there is no clear role is fundal pressure. This action does not alleviate a shoulder dystocia, because it simply duplicates the maternal expulsive force that already has failed to deliver the fetal shoulders. In addition, fundal pressure has been associated with both maternal (uterine rupture) and fetal (eg, spinal cord injury) injury.[1]

Although the maneuvers so far described are the ones most commonly performed, others also have been described. In the Gaskin maneuver, the patient is positioned onto her hands and knees and delivery is then attempted. This position has been reported to help with shoulder dystocia resolution. When a shoulder dystocia seems truly intractable and vaginal delivery does not seem possible, the operator may need to consider the performance of cephalic replacement (Zavanelli maneuver) and subsequent cesarean delivery. In the originally described Zavanelli maneuver, the head is rotated back to a prerestitution position, gently flexed, and then pushed back into the vagina with constant firm pressure. Tocolytic agents to relax the uterus may be considered in preparation for or during this maneuver. Other reported, but relatively rarely performed, techniques include symphysiotomy, intentional fetal clavicular fracture, and hysterotomy with abdominal rescue. Given that these maneuvers are inherently associated with maternal or fetal trauma, they should only be used in situations when other maneuvers cannot relieve the dystocia.

There is no consensus that a particular alleviating maneuver or sequence of alleviating maneuvers is preferred once a shoulder dystocia occurs. Two recent studies illustrate the lack of consistent evidence that one maneuver is preferred because it clearly leads to improved outcomes. In a retrospective observational study, Hoffman and colleagues[21] evaluated outcomes for 2018 women with a vertex fetus beyond 34 0/7 weeks of gestation who incurred a shoulder dystocia during the process of delivery. The investigators found that delivery of the posterior shoulder was the maneuver that was associated with the highest rate of delivery when compared with other maneuvers (84.4% compared with 24.3%–72.0%; $P<.005$–$P<.001$) and that it did not seem to result in any higher chance of neonatal injury (8.4% compared with 6.1%–14.0%; $P = .23$–$P = .07$). In contrast, Leung and colleagues[22] performed a study that resulted in a different conclusion. In their population, after McRoberts maneuver was not initially successful, rotational methods and posterior arm delivery were found to be similarly successful (72.0% vs 63.6%), but the former was associated with less-frequent brachial plexus palsy (4.4% vs 21.4%) and humeral fracture (1.1% vs 7.1%). The contrasting results of these studies underscore that there is no one "best" maneuver that should be applied first or no specific sequence of maneuvers that should always be used, but instead, that providers should use the maneuvers, based on their own facility and the individual circumstances, that they think are most amenable to resolving the dystocia.

WHAT IS THE ROLE FOR SIMULATION IN MANAGEMENT OF SHOULDER DYSTOCIA?

Several characteristics of shoulder dystocia, as heretofore described, make it a particular challenge to manage effectively.

1. Relative infrequency
2. Subjective criterion for diagnosis
3. Unpredictability
4. Need for coordinated actions of multiple team members to perform alleviating maneuvers

Given these potential barriers to the effective management of shoulder dystocia, investigators have attempted to enhance care by using protocols and simulation training. Simulation refers to the re-creation of an actual event that has previously occurred or could potentially occur.[23] Use of simulation can enhance patient safety because procedures can be practiced and repeated without ever exposing providers or patients to harm. Simulation often has been studied in the context of obstetric emergencies such as shoulder dystocia and eclampsia. For these occurrences, simulation may be helpful not only for individuals at the start of their career but also for experienced professionals, who can maintain skills that they need to use during unpredictable and uncommon events.

Results of studies have illustrated that simulation may enhance several aspects of shoulder dystocia management, including performance of the maneuvers, communication among team members, and documentation. Deering and colleagues[24] performed a randomized trial in which residents were randomized either to training for shoulder dystocia with a birth simulator or to no training with a simulator. Those given the training were significantly more likely to use maneuvers in a timely and correct manner in a subsequent simulation. Furthermore, residents who underwent training scored more highly on measures of overall performance and preparedness, as judged by a blinded observer. Another group of investigators randomized medical students to a 30-minute hands-on training session using a simulator or to a 30-minute training session in which students witnessed others perform shoulder dystocia management on a pelvic training model.[25] After 3 days, the skills of participants with regard to shoulder dystocia management were evaluated. Those who had undergone hands-on training were judged by others to have significantly better management skills, and these participants judged themselves to be more self-assured in their management.

Goffman and colleagues[26] studied outcomes after simulation training, not in medical students, but in residents and attending physicians. In their study, participants underwent a simulation of a shoulder dystocia followed by a debriefing that included (1) a brief lecture about shoulder dystocia, (2) a review of the basic maneuvers and a basic algorithm for management of shoulder dystocia, (3) a discussion of approaches that optimize team performance during an emergency, (4) a review of the key components of documentation, (5) a review of the digital recording of the simulations, and (6) a discussion of provider performance. During a subsequent shoulder dystocia simulation, resident and attending physicians demonstrated significant improvements in use of maneuvers, communication, and overall performance. Crofts and colleagues[27] obtained similar results in their multicenter study. These investigators randomized participants to partake in either a high-fidelity simulation (ie, using a mannequin with a high degree of biofidelity) or a low-fidelity simulation (eg, using a simple doll-like mannequin) and then reevaluated participants' performance during a simulated shoulder dystocia after the randomized simulation training. Some measures of performance (eg, total applied force) were improved to a greater extent in clinicians who had undergone high-fidelity simulation training, but many other outcomes (eg, magnitude of peak force, frequency of use of maneuvers) were similar between the 2 groups. It should be noted, however, that in none of the studies discussed so far were actual clinical outcomes evaluated. Accordingly, it cannot be known from these studies whether a simulation program will inevitably result in fewer brachial plexus palsies among women with shoulder dystocias.

Although studies of actual clinical outcomes are limited, there is some evidence that a program of shoulder dystocia simulation may be associated with fewer transient brachial plexus palsies. Draycott and colleagues[28] studied the outcomes associated with the introduction of a mandatory shoulder dystocia simulation for personnel on a labor and delivery unit in the United Kingdom. The frequency of transient brachial plexus palsy associated with a shoulder dystocia was significantly lower after providers underwent simulation training (7.4%–2.3%; risk ratio [RR], 0.31; 95% CI, 0.13–0.72).[18] MacKenzie and colleagues[29] also studied deliveries in the United Kingdom and found that management of shoulder dystocia improved after training. However, the frequency of brachial plexus palsy at the time of shoulder dystocia actually increased during the time of the study.

The results of other investigations of transient brachial plexus palsy in the United States have been more consistent with the results of Draycott and colleagues.[28] Inglis and colleagues[30] studied the frequency of brachial plexus palsy at their institution over 9 years. During this time, a shoulder dystocia protocol and training with a simulated shoulder dystocia were introduced. The frequency of brachial plexus palsy associated with shoulder dystocia, which was 30% at baseline, decreased to 10.7% after implementation of the protocol and simulation program (P<.01).

Before developing their shoulder dystocia protocol, Grobman and colleagues[31] explored the components of communication that providers think are important for a team to incorporate during a shoulder dystocia. In this study, 27 providers, drawn from the multidisciplinary team that contributes to obstetric care on a labor and delivery unit, were interviewed during a 2-month period by a single individual. Interviewees, and nurses in particular, noted that the team of obstetric providers was not always collectively and simultaneously aware that a shoulder dystocia had been diagnosed. Once the care team was alerted to the occurrence of a shoulder dystocia, providers commented that they thought it was important to be able to efficiently summon assistance and additional personnel. Providers also noted that when additional staff did arrive, there was the potential for lack of role clarity. This situation was particularly noted with regard to nursing staff, who needed to perform multiple actions (including calling other staff, performing maneuvers, obtaining other requested resources, and documenting activities). Physician respondents, in particular, noted that during a shoulder dystocia their concentration was so focused on alleviating the dystocia that they could lose track of the duration, which they thought was important to know so that optimal management decisions could be made.

After the interviews, Grobman and colleagues[31] developed a shoulder dystocia protocol that incorporated specific solutions to the concerns that had been voiced. The first component of this protocol is the action that activates the rest of the protocol, namely, the unambiguous announcement by the delivery provider, on diagnosis, that a "shoulder dystocia is present." Once this statement is made, roles and actions of the team members are delineated. The delivery provider then focuses on directing the alleviating maneuvers, while the patient's primary nurse directs actions of her nursing colleagues. The primary nurse also summons other relevant staff (including nurses, anesthesiologists, additional obstetricians, and pediatricians) through a single emergency call system. During the dystocia, a nurse is charged with calling out, in 30-second intervals, the length of time that has elapsed after delivery of the fetal head. To facilitate this action and the accuracy of the response, the primary nurse routinely (ie, at all deliveries) marks the fetal monitoring strip at the time of the delivery of the head. The entirety of the protocol is presented in **Fig. 1**.

This protocol was introduced at multidisciplinary sessions to all labor and delivery staff through a low-fidelity simulation that involved only simulation of the team response, with an actress portraying a patient and no repetition of maneuvers or delivery using a model pelvis. After introduction of this protocol, there was a decline in the frequency of brachial plexus palsies diagnosed at delivery (10.1%–2.6%, $P = .03$) and at neonatal discharge (7.6%–1.3%, $P = .04$).[32]

Despite the evidence that shoulder dystocia protocols and simulations may be associated with a reduction in the frequency of transient brachial plexus palsies, there is at present a lack of information about the consequence with regard to permanent brachial plexus palsies. For example, after the introduction of their simulation program, Draycott and colleagues[28] did not discern a significant difference in brachial

OB provider
- Announce shoulder dystocia

Triggers RN response →

- Communicate with patient/family

- Direct nurses to perform maneuvers, as appropriate
  - McRoberts
  - Suprapubic pressure

- Perform secondary maneuvers, as necessary
  - Rotational
  - Deliver posterior arm

L&D nurses
- Nurse Announces her "lead"

- Employ **TEAM** approach:

  Time
  - Note delivery of head using fetal monitor event marker
  - Call out 30-second intervals

  Emergency call light button
  - "We have a shoulder in LDR # and need a nurse and a resident to assist."

  Activate shoulder dystocia page

  Perform **M**aneuvers

- Upon arrival, third nurse retrieves worksheet and acts as Documenter:
  - Observe & record key information

Fig. 1. Shoulder dystocia protocol. OB, obstetric; L&D, labor and delivery; RN, registered nurse. (*From* Grobman WA, Hornbogen A, Burke C, et al. Development and implementation of a team-centered shoulder dystocia protocol. Simul Healthc 2010;5:199–203; with permission.)

plexus palsies that persisted either at 6 months (RR, 0.28; 95% CI, 0.07–1.1) or 12 months (RR, 0.41; 95% CI, 0.1–1.77). Inglis and colleagues[30] and Grobman and colleagues[32] did not collect data even for this length of time, and thus it is unknown whether their protocols were associated with any alteration in the frequency of permanent brachial plexus palsies.

REFERENCES

1. American College of Obstetrician and Gynecologists. Shoulder dystocia. ACOG Practice Bulletin No. 40. Obstet Gynecol 2002;100:1045–50.
2. Beall MH, Spong C, McKay J, et al. Objective definition of shoulder dystocia: a prospective evaluation. Am J Obstet Gynecol 1998;179:934–7.
3. Gherman RB. Shoulder dystocia: an evidence-based evaluation of the obstetric nightmare. Clin Obstet Gynecol 2002;45:345–62.
4. Rouse DJ, Owen J, Goldenberg RL, et al. The effectiveness and costs of elective cesarean delivery for fetal macrosomia diagnosed by ultrasound. JAMA 1996; 276:1480–6.
5. Gherman RB, Ouzounian JG, Goodwin TM. Obstetrical maneuvers for shoulder dystocia and associated fetal morbidity. Am J Obstet Gynecol 1998;178:1126–30.
6. Torki M, Barton L, Miller DA, et al. Severe brachial plexus palsy in women without shoulder dystocia. Obstet Gynecol 2012;120:539–41.
7. Dildy GA, Clark SL. Shoulder dystocia: risk identification. Clin Obstet Gynecol 2000;43:265–82.
8. Grobman WA, Stamilio DM. Methods of clinical prediction. Am J Obstet Gynecol 2006;194:888–94.
9. Nesbitt TS, Gilbert WM, Herrchen B. Shoulder dystocia and associated risk factors with macrosomic infants born in California. Am J Obstet Gynecol 1998; 179:476–80.
10. Dodd JM, Catcheside B, Scheil W. Can shoulder dystocia be reliably predicted? Aust N Z J Obstet Gynaecol 2012;52:248–52.
11. Lewis DF, Raymond RC, Perkins MB, et al. Recurrence rate of shoulder dystocia. Am J Obstet Gynecol 1995;172:1369–71.
12. Colombara DV, Soh JD, Menacho LA, et al. Birth injury in a subsequent vaginal delivery among women with a history of shoulder dystocia. J Perinat Med 2011;39:709–15.
13. Chauhan SP, Grobman WA, Gherman RA, et al. Suspicion and treatment of the macrosomic fetus: a review. Am J Obstet Gynecol 2005;193:332–46.
14. American College of Obstetrician and Gynecologists. Fetal macrosomia. ACOG Practice Bulletin 22. Washington, DC: ACOG; 2000.
15. Gonen O, Rosen DJ, Dolfin Z, et al. Induction of labor versus expectant management in macrosomia: a randomized study. Obstet Gynecol 1997;89:913–7.
16. Gonen R, Bader D, Ajami M. Effects of a policy of elective cesarean delivery in cases of suspected fetal macrosomia on the incidence of brachial plexus injury and the rate of cesarean delivery. Am J Obstet Gynecol 2000;183:1296–300.
17. Gherman RB, Tramont J, Muffley P, et al. Analysis of McRoberts' maneuver by X-ray pelvimetry. Obstet Gynecol 2000;95:43–7.
18. Beall MH, Spong CY, Ross MG. A randomized controlled trial of prophylactic maneuvers to reduce head-to-body delivery time in patients at risk for shoulder dystocia. Obstet Gynecol 2003;102:31–5.
19. Poggi SH, Spong CY, Allen RH. Prioritizing posterior arm delivery during severe shoulder dystocia. Obstet Gynecol 2003;101:1068–72.

20. Paris AE, Greenberg JA, Ecker JL, et al. Is an episiotomy necessary with a shoulder dystocia? Am J Obstet Gynecol 2011;205:217.e1–3.
21. Hoffman MK, Bailit JL, Brance DW, et al. A comparison of obstetric maneuvers for the acute management of shoulder dystocia. Obstet Gynecol 2011;117:1272–8.
22. Leung TY, Suart O, Suen SS, et al. Comparison of perinatal outcomes of shoulder dystocia alleviated by different type and sequence of manoeuvres: a retrospective review. BJOG 2011;118:985–90.
23. Hunt EA, Shilkofski NA, Atavroudis TA, et al. Simulation: translation to improved team performance. Anesthesiol Clin 2007;25:301–19.
24. Deering S, Poggi S, Macedonia C, et al. Improving resident competency in the management of shoulder dystocia with simulation training. Obstet Gynecol 2004;103:1224–8.
25. Buerkle B, Pueth J, Hefler LA, et al. Objective structured assessment of technical skills evaluation of theoretical compared with hands-on training of shoulder dystocia management: a randomized controlled trial. Obstet Gynecol 2012; 120:809–14.
26. Goffman D, Heo H, Pardanani S, et al. Improving shoulder dystocia management among resident and attending physicians using simulations. Am J Obstet Gynecol 2008;199:294.e1–5.
27. Crofts JF, Bartlett C, Ellis D, et al. Training for shoulder dystocia: a trial of simulation using low-fidelity and high-fidelity mannequins. Obstet Gynecol 2006;108: 1477–85.
28. Draycott TJ, Crofts JF, Ash JP, et al. Improving neonatal outcome through practical shoulder dystocia training. Obstet Gynecol 2008;112:14–20.
29. MacKenzie IZ, Shah M, Lean K, et al. Management of shoulder dystocia. Trends in incidence and maternal and neonatal mortality. Obstet Gynecol 2007;110: 1059–68.
30. Inglis SR, Feier N, Chetiyaar JB, et al. Effects of shoulder dystocia training on the incidence of brachial plexus injury. Am J Obstet Gynecol 2011;204:322.e1–6.
31. Grobman WA, Hornbogen A, Burke C, et al. Development and implementation of a team-centered shoulder dystocia protocol. Simul Healthc 2010;5:199–203.
32. Grobman WA, Miller D, Burke C, et al. Outcomes associated with introduction of a shoulder dystocia protocol. Am J Obstet Gynecol 2011;205:513–7.

Maternal Sepsis

Jamie Morgan, MD*, Scott Roberts, MD, MSc

KEYWORDS

- Maternal sepsis • Pyelonephritis • Pneumonia • Septic abortion

KEY POINTS

- The focus of this article is on sepsis related to simple maternal systemic inflammatory response syndrome.
- In developed countries, maternal sepsis is usually the result of puerperal sepsis and urinary tract infections.
- Labor and delivery units should focus on developing procedures that recognize unstable septic gravidas to ensure prompt recognition and appropriate therapies.

Maternal sepsis is relatively common. Most of these infections are the result of tissue damage during labor and delivery and physiologic changes normally occurring during pregnancy. Instigating organisms are usually from the polymicrobial flora of the genito-urinary tract. Common nonobstetric infections, which are often exacerbated by altered pregnancy physiology, also make a significant contribution to infectious morbidity in pregnancy. These infections, whether directly pregnancy-related or simply aggravated by normal pregnancy physiology, ultimately have the potential to progress to severe sepsis and septic shock. This article discusses commonly encountered entities and septic shock. Emphasized are the expeditious recognition of common maternal sepsis and meticulous attention to appropriate management to prevent the progression to severe sepsis and septic shock. Also discussed are principles and new approaches for the management of septic shock.

Obstetricians are lucky; their patients are generally young and healthy. Regardless, sepsis is not uncommon. It is more prevalent in developing nations where there are higher rates of HIV and malaria and less access to prenatal care.[1] In developed countries, such as the United States, maternal sepsis is usually the result of puerperal sepsis and urinary tract infections.[2] For purposes of clarity, definition, and comparison standardized definitions were published in 2003, shown in **Table 1**.[3]

Pregnancy predisposes women to four specific infectious complications: (1) pyelonephritis; (2) chorioamnionitis (often after cesarean delivery); (3) septic abortion; and (4) pneumonia. Sample rates of endometritis after vaginal birth (5%, 0%–24%) are

Maternal-Fetal Medicine, University of Texas Southwestern Medical Center, 5323 Harry Hines Boulevard, Dallas, TX 75390, USA
* Corresponding author.
E-mail address: jamie.morgan@utsouthwestern.edu

Obstet Gynecol Clin N Am 40 (2013) 69–87
http://dx.doi.org/10.1016/j.ogc.2012.11.007
0889-8545/13/$ – see front matter © 2013 Elsevier Inc. All rights reserved.

obgyn.theclinics.com

Table 1 Definition of terms	
	Presence of Microorganisms in a Normally Sterile Site
Bacteremia	Cultivatable bacteria in the bloodstream
Systemic inflammatory response syndrome	The systemic response to a wide range of stresses. Currently used criteria include two or more of the following: Temperature >38°C or <36°C Heart rate >90 beats/min Respiratory rate >20 breaths/min or $Paco_2$ <32 mm Hg White blood count >12,000 cells/mm³ or <4000 cells/mm³, or >10% immature (band) forms A potentially misleading term. The evidence that the body's early responses to infection cause systemic inflammation is controversial.
Sepsis	The systemic response to infection. If associated with proved or clinically suspected infection, systemic inflammatory response syndrome is called sepsis in the American consensus scheme.
Hypotension	A systolic blood pressure of <90 mm Hg, mean arterial pressure <70 mm Hg, or a reduction of >40 mm Hg from baseline.
Severe sepsis	Sepsis associated with dysfunction of organs distant from the site of infection, hypoperfusion, or hypotension. The term sepsis syndrome had a similar definition.
Septic shock	Sepsis with hypotension that despite adequate fluid resuscitation requires pressor therapy. In addition, there are perfusion abnormalities that may include lactic acidosis, oliguria, altered mental status, and acute lung injury.

lower than those undergoing nonelective cesarean (28.6%, 3%–61%).[4] If one adds in the rates of pyelonephritis, sepsis is not at all uncommon. Pyelonephritis accounts for 3% to 4% of all antepartum admissions[5] and makes up the largest proportion of the overall rare obstetric cases complicated by severe septic shock in the United States.[6,7] In obstetrics, this is not a common event. Clinicians prevent septic shock by appropriately treating sepsis. This should be the main goal. This article approaches the treatment of sepsis and discusses early goal directed therapy (EGDT) of septic shock to optimize outcomes and minimize maternal morbidity and mortality. Two excellent reviews of this latter subject have been recently published and are recommended.[8,9]

Because of the polymicrobial nature of puerperal sepsis (**Box 1**) and the gram-negative nature of upper urinary tract infection, it is important to know classes and combinations of antibiotics that treat these different kinds of infections (**Box 2**). **Box 3** lists different kinds of sepsis that are encountered and are representatively discussed.

PYELONEPHRITIS

Acute pyelonephritis is the most common severe medical complication of pregnancy and is the leading cause of septic shock in the pregnant patient.[7] The increased incidence of renal infection in pregnant patients compared with nonpregnant women is related to the relative obstruction of the urinary tract resulting from pregnancy physiology, dilation of the ureters secondary to progesterone and lack of protective peristalsis, and mechanical compression of the urinary system by the gravid uterus in conjunction with bacteriuria.[10] Low socioeconomic status is the most important risk

---

Box 1
Organisms involved with maternal sepsis

Gram-positive cocci

    Pneumococcus

    Streptococcus A and B

    Enterococcus faecalis

    Staphylococcus aureus

Gram-negative rods

    Escherichia coli

    Haemophilus influenza

    Klebsiella

    Enterobacter spp

    Proteus spp

    Pseudomonas spp

    Serratia spp

Gram-positive rods

    Listeria monocytogenes

Anaerobes

    Bacteroides spp

    Prevotella

    Clostridium perprfringens

    Fusobacterium spp

    Peptococcus

    Peptostreptococcus

Fungal species

Viral organisms

    Herpes and varicella

    HIV

    Influenza A and B

---

factor cited in the development of all urinary tract infections in pregnancy, and hence it is an exceedingly common diagnosis among medically indigent patients.[10]

The disease most commonly presents after the first trimester with fever, lumbar pain, shaking chills, nausea, and vomiting. On examination, costovertebral angle tenderness is generally noted and laboratory findings include microscopic bacteriuria and pyuria on urinalysis verified by a positive urine culture.[11] Fetal tachycardia can also be seen depending on the degree of maternal pyrexia. Normal bowel flora is the most commonly isolated organisms, with 70% to 80% of cases arising from *Escherichia coli* infection.[12] *Klebsiella*, *Proteus*, and *Enterobacter* account for most of the remaining cases, although a small number are caused by group B and enterococcal streptococci.

Box 2
Prevalent antibiotics used in maternal sepsis

Gold standards

  Clindamycin and gentamicin ± ampicillin

    Routine

  Vancomycin and zosyn

    Failure routine

Cephalosporins

  Cefoxitin (second generation)

  Cefotetan (second generation)

  Effective gram positive, gram negative, and anaerobes

  Cefotaxime (third generation)

  Ceftriaxone (third generation)

  More effective gram negative and some gram positive

Penicillin/β-lactamase inhibitors

  Unasyn

  Timentin

  Zosyn

Carbepenams

  Imepenam/cilistatin

  Meropenam

  Vancomycin

Hospitalization is generally recommended after the diagnosis of acute pyelonephritis given the risk of associated complications and 15% to 20% incidence of bacteremia. Empiric treatment is initiated with ampicillin plus gentamycin, a cephalosporin, or extended-spectrum penicillin. In most cases, appropriate antibiotic therapy in addition to aggressive intravenous hydration leads to rapid clinical improvement within 48 to 72 hours. However, up to one-fourth of women with severe infection have evidence of multiorgan derangement.[12]

Failure to respond to first-line antibiotic treatment within 72 hours should prompt evaluation for obstructive urinary tract lesions, such as urinary calculi and intrarenal or perinephric abscesses, which often lead to continuing urosepsis without further intervention. Endotoxin-mediated renal dysfunction with depressed glomerular filtration rate and hematologic abnormalities, such as anemia and thrombocytopenia, are relatively common complications of renal infection. Less commonly, acute pyelonephritis can result in respiratory insufficiency, which occurs in 1 in 50 women with severe infection.[13] Alveolar-capillary membrane permeability is altered by endotoxin release leading to pulmonary edema, which is transient and responds to supplemental oxygen in most women; however, in rare cases, the alveolar damage can lead to life-threatening respiratory distress syndrome.[14]

The most uncommon complication of acute pyelonephritis is septic shock. It is clinically important to distinguish between true septic shock defined by persistent

> **Box 3**
> **Different causes of maternal sepsis**
>
> Chorioamnionitis
> Metritis
> Septic abortion
> Pelvic abscess
> Septic pelvic thrombophlebitis
> Pneumonia
> Influenza A and B
>   Secondary infection
> Herpes
> Varicella
> Wound infection
> Necrotizing cellulitis
> Necrotizing fasciitis
> Appendicitis
> Cholecystitis
> Pancreatitis
> Small bowel injury

hypotension and diminished perfusion despite adequate fluid resuscitation as opposed to transient hypotension caused by hypovolemia, fever, anorexia, and vomiting. Women with septic shock syndrome (capillary endothelial damage, diminished vascular resistance, and low cardiac output) usually require intensive care often aided by the use of vasopressors to maintain adequate tissue perfusion.

Early presentation to prenatal care is essential to prevent the development of kidney infection, urosepsis, and septic shock. American College of Obstetricians and Gynecologists and the United States Preventive Task Force Services recommend screening for asymptomatic bacteriuria at the first prenatal visit.[15,16] Because urosepsis makes up one of the most common causes of septic shock and obstetric admissions to the intensive care unit (ICU), the implementation of judicious screening and treatment policies should make this devastating complication even rarer.

CHORIOAMNIONITIS

Chorioamnionitis or intra-amniotic infection refers to acute inflammation of the chorion, amnion, and placenta. Clinical chorioamnionitis typically results from ascending polymicrobial infection in the setting of rupture of membranes; however, it can occur with intact membranes and also can rarely result from hematogenous spread or invasive procedures. Overall, chorioamnionitis complicates 1% to 4% of term deliveries in the United States and 5% to 10% of preterm deliveries.[17,18] Risk factors associated with intra-amniotic infection include young age, prolonged labor, nulliparity, prolonged rupture of membranes, multiple vaginal examinations, meconium-stained amniotic fluid, internal monitoring, group B streptococcus colonization, and bacterial vaginosis. Ascending infection from the lower genital tract leads to a polymicrobial intra-amniotic infection. The genital mycoplasmas, *Ureaplasma urealyticum* and *Mycoplasma hominis*, are the most commonly isolated organisms in culture-confirmed chorioamnionitis, occurring in up to 47% and 30% of cases, respectively.[19,20] Other commonly implicated microbes include anaerobes, such as *Gardnerella vaginalis* and *Bacteriodes*; group B streptococcus; and gram-negative rods, such as *E coli*.

Clinical chorioamnionitis, as the name suggests, is diagnosed solely based on clinical signs. Various diagnostic criteria are used, but the authors typically use a temperature greater than 100.4°F intrapartum to make the diagnosis. Patients with preterm rupture being expectantly managed sometimes display uterine tenderness with the development of infection. Management of patients with intra-amniotic infection involves initiation of broad-spectrum antibiotics and delivery. The most widely used regimen is intravenous administration of ampicillin every 6 hours and gentamycin dosed every 8 to 24 hours (coverage for group B streptococcus and *E coli*); clindamycin or metronidazole is added to the regimen for anaerobic coverage in the setting of cesarean delivery. Multiple studies have demonstrated that immediate intrapartum administration of antibiotics reduces maternal and fetal complications compared with immediate postpartum treatment.[21,22]

The prognosis for women diagnosed with chorioamnionitis is generally good; however, intra-amniotic infection does increase the likelihood of labor abnormalities and leads to a twofold to threefold increased risk of cesarean section. It also increases the risk for wound infection, pelvic abscess, and postpartum hemorrhage. Maternal bacteremia is an uncommon consequence of intra-amniotic infection and occurs in less than 10% of cases.[23] However, more serious complications, such as septic shock, disseminated intravascular coagulation, adult respiratory distress syndrome, and maternal death, may occur but are exceedingly rare. Nevertheless, chorioamnionitis should be promptly recognized and treated because it can lead to devastating neonatal consequences, including fetal bacteremia, clinical sepsis, and fetal death.

SEPTIC ABORTION

The occurrence of septic abortion is now rare in the United States. Antibiotic prophylaxis with surgical abortion has helped reduce the rate of septic abortion since its application in the mid-1990s.[24] After March 2006, and several clostridial-related deaths after medical abortion (abortion by means of medication), the Planned Parenthood Association of America required that providers either screen patients for chlamydia and gonorrhea (if living in endemic areas) and treat, or supply doxycycline prophylaxis with medically induced abortion. The rate of serious infection after medical abortion declined with the institution of prophylactic antibiotics and the switch from vaginal to buccal misoprostol.[25] Regardless, septic abortion remains a serious cause of maternal sepsis and ICU admissions.[26–28]

Sepsis related to septic abortion is mediated through metritis. Occasionally paraendometritis, peritonitis, and endocarditis are involved. After the diagnosis of septic abortion is established, treatment with broad-spectrum antibiotics should be immediately instituted. Simultaneously, evaluation for and removal of any retained products of conception should occur to prevent the development of sepsis. Rarely, hysterectomy in addition to oophorectomy may be required if a dusky, devitalized uterus or pelvic tissue crepitus is encountered intraoperative and clostridial infection is suspected.[29] Sepsis development is heralded by tachycardia, tachypnea, hypotension, and hyperthermia or hypothermia. In cases of clostridial infection, exotoxin release can lead to the development of toxic shock syndrome. Toxin release leads to vascular permeability, massive fluid leakage, body cavity effusions, and resultant organ failure.[30] Patients generally present within 2 to 7 days postabortion with nonspecific symptoms, such as nausea, vomiting, and abdominal pain, which can rapidly progress to refractory hypotension with multiorgan failure secondary to massive capillary leakage.[31] Interestingly, affected individuals do not develop fever with this anaerobic etiology. Regardless of the infectious cause, supportive care in addition to prompt initiation of antibiotics is essential to prevent potential morbidity or mortality.

In general, most serious postabortion infectious complications can be avoided in modern medicine. The availability of safe and accessible abortion services in the United States is essential to maintaining a low postabortion infection rate. Additionally, women presenting with signs and symptoms of infection after abortion procedures require prompt evaluation and management to avoid septic complications.

ENDOMETRITIS

The term "postpartum endometritis" encompasses a spectrum of infections including infection of the endometrial lining, the myometrium, and the parametrium.[32] It represents a fairly common puerperal complication. Mode of delivery is the most important risk factor for ultimate development of pelvic infection.[10] Other risk factors include labor and ruptured membranes. Endometritis originates from bacterial ascension from the lower genital tract during the labor process. Bacteria then colonize the decidua and amniotic fluid, but the infection does not become clinically apparent until after delivery.

Generally, these infections are polymicrobial. Common pathogens include anaerobic and aerobic bacteria, with 60% to 70% of cases involving both aerobes and anaerobes.[33] *Peptostreptococcus*, *Bacteriodes*, and *Clostridium* spp are typical anaerobic organisms and causative aerobes include group B streptococcus, enterococcus, and *E coli*. The presence of hematomas or devitalized tissue promotes bacterial growth, particularly of more virulent bacteria, such as *Streptococcus pyogenes* or *Staphylococcus aureus*. Diagnosis is usually clinical and fever is the most important criterion to suggest the diagnosis. Tachycardia, uterine or parametrial tenderness, and foul smelling lochia or purulent vaginal discharge helps to confirm the diagnosis of endometritis. Most fevers that do occur after delivery are secondary to genital tract infection. In women who undergo vaginal delivery and subsequently become febrile, only about 20% are ultimately diagnosed with a pelvic infection; however, in postoperative cesarean delivery patients, 70% of those who become febrile are diagnosed with a pelvic infection.[34]

Treatment of endometritis involves intravenous therapy with broad-spectrum antibiotics. The most commonly used combination is clindamycin and gentamycin, which has a 95% response rate.[35] Because many enterococcal infections are not responsive to this initial therapy, ampicillin is often added either primarily or after 48 to 72 hours if clinical response is poor.[36] Other antibiotic regimens involve extended-spectrum penicillin–β-lactamase inhibitor combinations or extended-spectrum cephalosporins. In more than 90% of women, broad-spectrum antibiotic regimens lead to improvement within 48 to 72 hours; however, if no improvement is seen within 72 hours, imaging studies should generally be undertaken to search for a fluid collection or surgical site inflammation.

Endometritis has the potential to result in more severe infectious morbidities, which often manifest in the form of persistent pyrexia. Generalized peritonitis may result from endometritis complicated by uterine incisional necrosis or dehiscence. In women who develop endometritis after cesarean delivery, parametrial cellulitis with phlegmon formation in the broad ligament may lead to persistent fever. Rarely, a parametrial phlegmon may suppurate forming a pelvic abscess, which requires direct or computed tomography–guided drainage. If the abscess ruptures, peritonitis develops and initial symptoms are those of adynamic ileus. Finally, postpartum pelvic infections can spread along the venous channels, causing thrombosis and leading to septic pelvic thrombophlebitis. This responds well to continued broad-spectrum antibiotic therapy.[37]

Endometritis is a common diagnosis with the potential for significant morbidity and even mortality, including prolonged hospitalization, wound disruption, and even peripartum hysterectomy for uterine necrosis and refractory infection. Aside from septic shock, this may be the most destructive sequela to the patient. A preventive measure recently used by American College of Obstetricians and Gynecologists and obstetricians around the United States is preoperative prophylactic antibiotics with cesarean sections.[38]

WOUND INFECTION AND *STREPTOCOCCUS PYOGENES* (GROUP A STREP)

According to the Centers for Disease Control and Prevention, surgical site infections (SSI) are the second most common health care–associated infection.[39] SSI are divided into superficial and deep, depending on which abdominal wall layers are involved, with the former involving the skin and subcutaneous tissue of the incision and the latter affecting the muscle and fascial layers of the abdominal wall. To qualify as a SSI, the infection must manifest within 30 days of the procedure in association with purulent wound drainage; wound cultures showing bacterial growth; or signs of infection at the wound site, such as redness, tenderness, and heat.[40]

As noted, the widespread use of prophylactic antibiotics before cesarean delivery has reduced the rate of postoperative infections; however, wound morbidity still remains a significant complication with the SSI rate ranging from 2% to 6% after cesarean section. Most of these wound infections come from unscheduled cesareans after women have labored with ruptured membranes.[41,42] Surgical risk factors, such as increased blood loss and longer operative times, increase the chance of infection. Multiple host factors, such as obesity, diabetes, hypertension, anemia, immunosuppression, smoking, and lower socioeconomic status, also contribute to postoperative wound morbidity. Most SSIs derive from a patient's endogenous vaginal micoflora and are usually polymicrobial. Causative organisms include gram-positive and -negative bacteria and facultative and obligate anaerobes.

Wound infections are often diagnosed in patients who are persistently febrile being treated for postpartum endometritis; a developing incisional abscess should be considered in women with persistent fever beyond postoperative Day 4. The diagnosis is made based on temperature elevation and the physical examination findings of pain and tenderness around the wound site. Superficial SSIs involving the tissue skin and subcutaneous fat may manifest as cellulitis alone. If the wound edges remain well approximated and no fluid drainage is noted, antimicrobial treatment alone is often sufficient to treat the infection; however, if any purulent drainage is noted, the wound should be opened to facilitate drainage of pus. Necrotic material should be debrided, followed by frequent repacking of the defect with saline-moistened gauze. Systemic manifestations of sepsis may develop in more extensive infections, particularly if broad-spectrum antimicrobial treatment is not initiated promptly.

A deep SSI involves the fascia and muscle of the anterior abdominal wall. Infection of the fascia leads to fascial dehiscence with subsequent evisceration and hernia formation. The most common and severe manifestation of deep SSI is necrotizing fasciitis, which is generally a polymicrobial infection resulting in necrosis of all layers of the abdominal wall. Occasionally, necrotizing fasciitis results from infection from a single virulent bacterial species, such as group A β-hemolytic streptococcus or *S aureus*. Early necrotizing fasciitis is virtually indistinguishable from cellulitis. Late manifestations include severe pain, crepitus, bullae formation, wound drainage, and clinical signs of sepsis. The diagnosis can only be confirmed by surgical exploration. Treatment consists of broad-spectrum antimicrobial coverage and excision of all necrotic tissue. Although necrotizing fasciitis is uncommon, it has a high associated mortality rate and must be quickly recognized to avoid potentially devastating consequences.

Streptococcus pyogenes (group A streptococcus) is a gram-positive cocci whose sepsis-causing properties in the puerperium are well documented. The organism is enveloped in a thick hyaluronic acid capsule, which inhibits and slows phagocytosis by macrophages and leukocytes in the infected gravida. M protein is the major virulence factor of this organism and strains lacking it are not virulent. This filamentous macromolecule affixes to the cell membrane, and traverses and penetrates the cell wall. It exerts its antiphagocytic effect by inhibiting activation of the alternate complement pathway on the cell surface. Several adhesins play critical roles in the first steps of adherence to the surface of human epithelial cells. Streptolysin O and S are extracellular hemolysins, which are toxic to a variety of human cells. Streptococcal pyrogenic exotoxins are a family of exotoxins associated with streptococcal toxic shock syndrome and necrotizing fasciitis.

In the mid-1980s, clinicians began to see certain streptococcal strains causing life-threatening invasive infections in a frequency and severity not seen for decades. Strains isolated from these invasive subtypes were mostly of M types 1 and 3. In many cases these infections gave rise to shock and multiorgan failure. These features, previously recorded for staphylococcal toxic shock syndrome, earned these entities the term "strep toxic shock syndrome."

PUERPERAL MASTITIS

Puerperal mastitis is a fairly common and potentially dangerous form of maternal sepsis. Symptoms usually appear after the first week postpartum. It is usually unilateral, and marked engorgement usually precedes inflammation. Presentation includes chills and rigors, fever, and tachycardia. There is a thickening or hardening of the affected breast, erythema, and severe pain. *S aureus* is the most frequently isolated organism and the most dangerous. Suckling infants are the immediate source of these organisms. Cases of toxic shock syndrome secondary to mastitis are described.[43,44] Most concerning is the recent appearance of community-acquired methicillin-resistant *S aureus* (CA-MRSA).[45] Infants may be exposed to hospital-acquired MRSA in the nursery or in the community. About one-third of women hospitalized with mastitis develop breast abscess and most of these are caused by CA-MRSA.[46]

Assessment of the severity of infection is important. Usually, such antibiotics as oral dicloxacillin or intravenous nafcillin coupled with pumping of the breast are all that are required (erythromycin may be substituted for dicloxacillin if for penicillin allergy). However, the extent of inflammation and the degree of systemic response may require admission, hydration, and parenteral antibiotics. Breast abscess may require surgical incision and drainage or aspiration. Milk from the affected breast should be aspirated and sent for culture and sensitivity before treatment (anaerobic infections are extremely unusual). If inadequate response from the aforementioned treatment is forthcoming, methicillin resistance may be a problem, and vancomycin should be started. Of note, the authors have experience with CA-MRSA that has responded to nafcillin, incision and drainage, and breast pumping. In case current management that does not involve vancomycin therapy is working, it seems unnecessary to start this medication even with a report of methicillin resistance.[33] As in all cases of maternal sepsis, timely diagnosis and management prevent much more serious sequelae.

PNEUMONIA

Clinicians have come a long way since the rate of maternal mortality from pneumonia was 20%.[47] The incidence of pneumonia in pregnancy, a common infection of the pulmonary parenchyma, is about 0.5 to 1.5 per 1000 pregnancies in the United States.[48,49] This is not different from that of reproductive-aged women in the general population. What is different is the increased morbidity of pneumonia in pregnancy. This is generally attributed to decreased residual lung volume and the 20% to 25% increased oxygen consumption required to support the gestation. Also responsible is a loss of lower esophageal sphincter tone. All of these changes push the pregnant woman a little closer to the cliff of decompensation.

Most community-acquired pneumonia in pregnancy is bacterial (93%).[50] Some of the organisms that cause bacterial pneumonia are *Streptococcus pneumonia*, *Heamophilus influenzae*, *C Pneumoniae*, *Mycoplasma pneumonia*, and *Legionella pneumophilia*. These infections respond well to macrolides, such as erythromycin and azithromycin. Severe community-acquired pneumonia is defined by the criteria given in **Box 4**.[51] In addition to requiring a higher level of care, additional antibiotic coverage should be added to macrolide therapy, such as a second- or third-generation cephalosporin (β-lactam). Severe pneumonia can lead to acute respiratory distress syndrome requiring mechanical ventilation and severe sepsis and septic shock syndrome. Of note, chest radiographs may lag behind the actual clinical picture. Community-acquired methicillin *S aureus* can cause a necrotizing pneumonia or can be a super infection with influenza pneumonia.[52,53] In this setting, vancomycin (at least) should be added to oseltamivir therapy.

INFLUENZA

Influenza in pregnant women has historically been associated with a higher rate of morbidity and mortality. The Spanish Flu in 1918 killed 21 to 50 million people worldwide. The mortality rate in pregnant women was 27% to 45%.[54] Although the hope is

Box 4
Criteria for severe community acquired pneumonia
1. Respiratory rate >30/min
2. Pao_2/Fio_2 ratio <250
3. Multilobar infiltrates
4. Confusion and disorientation
5. Uremia
6. Leukopenia WBC <4000/μl
7. Thrombocytopenia platelets <100,000/μl
8. Hypothermia core temperature <36°C
9. Hypotension requiring aggressive fluid resuscitation

that the likes of this flu are not seen again, most clinicians believe it is not a matter of "if" but rather of "when." The disease is spread by respiratory droplets and is very infectious. Generally, patients are infectious 2 days before the onset of symptoms and for 5 days thereafter.

Presenting symptoms include cough, fever, malaise, rhinitis, myalgias, headache, chills, and sore throat. Less common symptoms include nausea and vomiting, otitis, and conjunctival burning. Signs include fever, tachycardia, facial flushing, clear nasal discharge, and cervical adenopathy. Generally, fever lasts for 3 days with resolution of symptoms within 1 week. A rapid test can detect Influenza A and B, but sensitivities differ seasonally. If suspicion is strong, culture should be performed. Initial presentation is of systemic inflammatory response syndrome (sepsis), but rapid diagnosis or suspicion, supportive treatment, and antivirals usually lead to amelioration of disease in a timely fashion. Oxygen, hydration, and oseltamivir (neuraminidase inhibitor) started immediately helps achieve this therapeutic goal.

Occasionally, complications ensue. In the H1N1 flu variant of 1918, the systemic response from immunocompetent gravidas (most healthy people) caused a lethal inflammatory response in the lungs. Damage to lung parenchyma led to massive pulmonary damage and insufficiency, and it was not unusual to see people healthy in the morning, dusky and dead by the late afternoon. In addition to early aggressive antiviral therapy, oxygen, and hydration, ventilation providing positive end expiratory pressure may be vital while the disease runs its course and resolves.

Occasionally, superimposed viral or bacterial pneumonia complicates influenza infection. If such is suspected, usually occurring 2 to 14 days after initiation of symptoms, therapy for complicated pneumonia should be started. Erythromycin and a β-lactam, such as ceftriaxone or cefuroxime, should be added. Severe cases of pneumonia can be complicated by septic shock, heart and renal failure, and acute respiratory distress syndrome; ICU consultation and admission should be affected.

APPENDICITIS

Appendicitis has been confirmed in approximately 1 in 1500 pregnancies.[55] Signs and symptoms lead surgeons to explore about 1 in 1000 pregnancies, so the positive predictive value of signs and symptoms is only about two-thirds. It is a difficult but extremely important diagnosis to make. Signs and symptoms are confounded by the nausea and vomiting inherent to pregnancy, the deflection of the appendix by the rising fundus, and the potentially unusual location of pain. As the fundus rises and deflects the pelvis, the omentum is less able to wall off a "hot" appendix. The incidence of perforation progressively increases during gestation with approximations of 8%, 12%, and 20% in successive trimesters. Diagnostic accuracy decreases as gestation progresses, probably because of anatomic differences with the rising fundus.

Persistent abdominal pain and tenderness are common. Fever and elevating white blood count also are present. The authors have found the best tool for diagnosis in the presence of these symptoms is appendiceal computed tomography.[56] If the diagnosis is strongly suspected or confirmed with imaging, intravenous fluids and broad-spectrum antibiotics are started, and appendectomy is performed. In the absence of perforation, the antibiotics are usually stopped quickly postoperative, but in the presence of perforation they must be continued. With perforation and abscess there may also be coincident septic shock with its subsequent morbidity.

The morbidity and mortality of appendicitis is increased in pregnancy.[57] This is usually from delayed diagnosis and subsequent complications of sepsis. It is important to pursue this diagnosis when symptoms appear.

CHOLECYSTITIS

The incidence of asymptomatic gallstones in pregnant women is 2.5% to 10%.[58] For symptomatic cholelithiasis, treatment includes oral bile acid therapy with ursodeoxycholic acid (Actigall); antispasmodics (dicyclomine); extracorporeal shock wave lithotripsy (not done during pregnancy); and surgical removal. Acute cholecystitis usually develops when there is obstruction of the cystic duct. Bacterial infection plays a role in 50% to 85% of cases. Acute disease is associated with right upper quadrant pain, anorexia, nausea and vomiting, low-grade fever, and mild leukocytosis.

During pregnancy approximately 1 in 1000 women develop cholecystitis. Pregnancy is lithogenic. Gall bladder volume during fasting and residual volume after contracting in response to a test meal are doubled. Incomplete emptying leads to stasis and an increased incidence of cholesterol gallstones. Usually medical therapy is instituted. This consists of nasogastric suction, intravenous fluids, antimicrobials, and analgesics instituted before surgical therapy. If conservative nonsurgical therapy is instituted, cholecystitis recurs more than 50% of the time.

Current management favors surgical management. Conservative management leads to an increased risk for preterm delivery. Most experts believe that laparoscopic cholecystectomy is safe throughout pregnancy.[59,60] Endoscopic retrograde cholangiopancreatography can relieve common duct stones. Complications from cholecystitis can lead to pancreatitis and severe sepsis. Again, prudent management, usually surgical, minimizes these problems.

TUBERCULOSIS

Widespread screening for tuberculosis (TB) should not be affected without cause. When clinically appropriate, screening protocols including tuberculin skin test or interferon-γ release assay test may be performed. The benefits of the latter are quick turnaround, less false positivity, and are not altered by previous testing because they are performed on blood from the individual to detect tuberculin immune response to white blood cells.

The following people should be tested for TB infection: people who have spent time with someone who has active TB disease; people with HIV infection or another medical problem that weakens the immune system; people with symptoms of TB disease (fever, night sweats, cough, and weight loss); people from a country where TB disease is common (most countries in Latin America, the Caribbean, Africa, Asia, Eastern Europe, and Russia); and people who use illegal drugs. Most TB is latent, but a certain percentage (5%–10%) may become active and lead to sepsis in certain situations.[61]

In young children with immature cell-mediated immunity and in persons with impaired immunity (eg, HIV infections and poor nutrition), primary pulmonary TB may progress rapidly to clinical illness. In the absence of an adequate acquired immune response, which usually contains the infection, disseminated or miliary disease may result. In order of frequency, the extrapulmonary sites most commonly involved in TB are the lymph nodes, pleura, genitourinary tract, bones, and joints, meninges, peritoneum, and pericardium. However, virtually all organ systems may be affected. As a result of hematogenous dissemination in individuals infected with HIV, extrapulmonary TB is seen more commonly today than in the past.

Even though tuberculin skin test or interferon-γ release assay testing are standard for HIV-infected gravidas, a chest radiograph also should be obtained. Many people advocate delaying treatment in gravidas until after delivery, but in the HIV-infected gravid population, the recommendation is to treat.[62,63] Latent TB proceeds to pulmonary TB in 8% of these cases (as opposed to 1%–2% in the general population). Isoniazid (INH) and pyridoxine for 9 months are standard for latent TB, but pulmonary and extrapulmonary disease is more common in this group and requires four-drug therapy (INH, rifampin, pyrazinamide, and ethambutol). With reconstitution of their immunity after several weeks of highly active antiretroviral therapy, it is not unusual to see paradoxic reactions caused by immune reconstitution. These reactions include hectic fevers; lymphadenopathy (sometimes severe); a worsening chest radiographic TB appearance (eg, miliary infiltrates, pleural effusion); and worsening of the original tuberculous lesions (cutaneous and peritoneal).

Extrapulmonary or miliary disease is much more common in parturients infected with HIV and the importance of underlying conditions, such as alcoholism, cirrhosis, neoplasm, pregnancy, rheumatologic disease, and treatment with immunosuppressive agents, cannot be overlooked. Generalized symptoms of fever, anorexia, weakness, and weight loss are nonspecific. Headache may indicate meningitis, abdominal pain may be caused by peritonitis, and pleural pain may result from pleuritis. Physical findings are likewise usually nonspecific, but a careful search for cutaneous eruptions, sinus tracts, and lymphadenopathy may yield a prompt biopsy diagnosis. A miliary infiltrate on chest roentgenogram is the most helpful finding and the usual reason miliary TB is suspected. Unfortunately, many patients, particularly the elderly, succumb to miliary TB before the chest roentgenogram becomes abnormal. If one suspects this type of illness in an immunocompromised pregnant woman, consult adult infectious disease to aid in therapy. Depending on the patient status, ICU care with ventilation, pressors, and oxygen support may be necessary.

SEVERE SEPSIS AND SEPTIC SHOCK

Septic shock is rare in pregnancy occurring in 2 to 10 per 100,000 deliveries.[9,64] Although rare, it was recently found to be the leading cause of maternal death in the United Kingdom, and most of these cases were related to group A streptococcal puerperal sepsis.[65] In a recent study from Argentina, septic abortion was the major pelvic infectious cause of maternal mortality, and believed to be related to illegal practices of abortion in this nonsecular country. It is believed that gram-negative urosepsis and influenza pneumonia with its sequelae are also major components of maternal septic shock and mortality.

When critical physiologic decompensation is pending, it is imperative to apply supportive techniques including mechanical ventilation, vasopressor, and volume resuscitation in a critical care environment. A multidisciplinary team must be activated. Unless one has obstetric intensivists at the hospital, there is a very good chance that medical ICU personnel (medical intensivists, pulmonary, cardiac, and nephrology) and surgery will become quickly involved. Critical features of the pregnant woman mandate that one stay involved. A good guideline is the following: as maternal health goes, so goes the fetal health. The temptation to deliver the baby must be resisted until maternal stability is ensured.

In a review of 51 pregnant patients who were mechanically ventilated at one institution over 9 years, 24 patients were delivered by cesarean. Eleven of these were for "maternal condition." The mortality rate among these individuals of 36% highlights the tremendous stress surgery places on the maternal condition. These authors concluded that obstetric, not maternal, conditions should dictate delivery timing and mode.[66]

CARDIOVASCULAR SUPPORT

The aim of cardiovascular support is to maintain adequate cardiac output and blood pressure. As noted, there is a 20% increase in maternal oxygen demand in pregnancy. Cardiac output increases by 30% to 50% because of an increased stroke volume and heart rate. Blood pressure is reduced by 5 to 10 mm Hg by mid pregnancy, mainly as a result of progesterone effects on smooth muscle in the vascular tree. There is little change in the central venous pressure and pulmonary capillary wedge pressure (PCWP) in pregnancy.[67]

Cardiovascular support is required in cases of septic shock. Inadequate perfusion leads to anaerobic metabolism, increased serum lactate, and decreased maternal central venous oxygen saturation (Svo_2). This affects fetal oxygenation and nonreassuring fetal heart rates will be seen. A lactate level higher than 2 mmol/L indicates tissue hypoxia. Serial lactate levels are useful in judging the patient's response to circulatory support.[68]

Colloid osmotic pressure (COP) is reduced during pregnancy from 28 to about 23 mm Hg.[69] This is caused by a normal decrease in albumin concentration during pregnancy.[70] Each gram of albumin per deciliter exerts about 6 mm Hg pressure. The COP-PCWP gradient is usually about 8 mm Hg. As it decreases, the chance for pulmonary edema increases. With damage to pulmonary endothelium from endotoxins or exotoxins, a leak of protein across membranes occurs, leading to an even further decrease in the COP-PCWP gradient. Capillary and alveolar damage can lead to alveolar flooding and pulmonary edema even with low or normal capillary wedge pressures. If the damage continues, progression to acute respiratory distress syndrome may occur. This underlines the importance of rapid volume support and institution of broad-spectrum antibiotic therapy. The longer inflammation from microbial by-products remains unchecked, the more serious is end organ (eg, lung) damage.

Knowledge that pregnancy is a state of hypervolemia is helpful. Albumin concentrations seem low because that is the normal state in pregnancy. Colloid infusion is not recommended over crystalloid. Confounding treatment of sepsis with unproved (and unsafe) tocolytic protocols is not helpful. One should try to imagine under which circumstance surgery or chemical induction for delivery helps the septic patient, and then make sure it is achieved.

Early signs of decompensation include vasodilation with compensatory baroreceptor stimulated tachycardia. As cardiac output increases the renin-angiotensin system activates attempting to maintain vascular tone and increase intravascular volume. Goal-directed therapy suggests keeping the mean arterial pressure at 65 to 90 mm Hg. At less than 50 mm Hg the use of vasopressors is suggested. Sometimes it is necessary to give several liters of normal saline to achieve this goal.[71]

Pregnancy is a procoagulant state. In gram-negative sepsis (the main actor in urosepsis), endotoxin is released from lysed bacteria. This activates the coagulation cascade and inhibits the fibrinolytic system. Microthrombi are formed and damage the renal glomeruli. Hemolysis is mediated by endotoxin and may require transfusion. Direct hemolysis may occur from streptococcal or staphylococcal exotoxins.

It is not certain that elevated coagulation parameters (eg, prothrombin time, international normalized ratio) should be corrected in the absence of bleeding.[72] Platelets should be replaced with counts less than 5000/mm^3 and between 5 and 30,000/mm^3 if there is significant bleeding risk.[73,74] Another marker of tissue hypoxia is lactate. A

Box 5
Early goal-directed therapy

1. Blood cultures before antibiotic administration

2. Measure serum lactate levels

3. Broad-spectrum antibiotics started within 1 hour

4. Placement of central venous and arterial catheters

5. 500-mL bolus of crystalloid every 30 minutes to achieve a central venous pressure of 8–12 mm Hg

6. If mean arterial pressure <65, vasopressors given

7. If mean arterial pressure >90, vasodilators given

8. If $Scvo_2$ <70%, red cells transfused to achieve a hematocrit of 30%

9. Maintain urine output of 0.5 mL/kg/h

---

tissue lactate of greater than 4 mmol/L correlates with extensive tissue hypoxia, anaerobic metabolism from underperfused tissues, and a diagnosis of severe sepsis. Early lactate clearance has been associated with improved outcome in severe sepsis and septic shock.

EGDT has been promoted in the treatment of severe sepsis and septic shock as to providing significant benefit with respect to outcomes. There are no prospective studies in patients who are pregnant or postpartum concerning this approach (or any other management protocol for that matter). Rivers and coworkers[71] landmark trial provided early goals for severe sepsis and septic shock and is illustrated in **Box 5**. A major challenge to implementing EGDT is the protocol itself. It is complex and must be effected immediately. $Scvo_2$ monitoring is expensive; requires placement of central lines; and these requirements place a burden on medical areas (eg, labor and delivery and obstetric recovery rooms) that usually accept sick pregnant patients. Even with significant efforts and training in ICUs (medical ICUs), full implementation of EGDT has been poor.[75]

As an alternative for the obstetrician, a process developed in the United Kingdom called the "Sepsis Six" may be a more realistic goal in front-line management as multidisciplinary teams are mobilized.[76,77] This process is listed in **Box 6**. It has been associated with improved outcomes and is much easier for an unprepared unit (at least as to the extent demanded by EGDT) to implement.[78] This adds the need for oxygen therapy and accurate urine output monitoring.

Box 6
The sepsis six: to be delivered within 1 hour

1. High-flow oxygen applied

2. Blood and other relevant cultures

3. Administer broad-spectrum antibiotics

4. Measure serum lactate or alternative

5. Start IV fluid resuscitation with crystalloids

6. Accurate urine output measurement

SUMMARY

There is more concern with the treatment of simple maternal systemic inflammatory response syndrome–related sepsis in this article. The intricacies of inflammatory mechanisms producing the severe sepsis and septic shock picture are avoided. There is much concern with recognition of treatment failures of common obstetric infectious complications that occasionally turn into severe sepsis and septic shock. Mortality from these syndromes is unacceptably high. In one of the very few series on the subject, the rate of maternal mortality from sepsis and shock was 28%.[7] Labor and delivery units and their respective hospitals should strive to develop processes that ensure that unstable septic gravidas receive prompt recognition and appropriate therapies. Specific examples of these processes (eg, EGDT) are currently being tested in national and international trials.[79]

REFERENCES

1. Dolea C, Stein S. Global burden of maternal sepsis in the year 2000. Evidence and information for policy (EIP). Geneva (Switzerland): World Health Organization; 2003.
2. Maupin RT. Obstetric infection disease emergencies. Clin Obstet Gynecol 2002; 45:393–404.
3. American College of Chest Physicians/Society of Critical Care Medicine. Consensus Conference definitions for sepsis and organ failure and guidelines for the use of innovative therapies in sepsis. Crit Care Med 1992;20: 864–74.
4. Smaill F, Hofmeyer GJ. Antibiotic prophylaxis for cesarean section. Cochrane Database Syst Rev 2002;(3):CD000933.
5. Jamieson DJ, Schiid L, Adams MM, et al. Hospitalizations during pregnancy among managed care enrollees. Obstet Gynecol 2002;100(1):94–100.
6. Lee W, Clark SL, Cotton DB, et al. Septic shock during pregnancy. Am J Obstet Gynecol 1988;159:410–6.
7. Mabie WC, Barton JR, Sibai B. Septic shock in pregnancy. Obstet Gynecol 1997; 90:553–61.
8. Guinn DA, Abel DE, Tomlinson MW. Early goal directed therapy for sepsis during pregnancy. Obstet Gynecol Clin North Am 2007;34:459–79.
9. Barton JR, Sibai S. Severe sepsis and septic shock in pregnancy. Obstet Gynecol 2012;120:689–706.
10. Cunningham G, Leveno K, Bloom S, et al. Williams obstetrics. 23rd edition. New York: McGraw-Hill; 2010.
11. Gilstrap LC, Ramen S. Urinary tract infections during pregnancy. Obstet Gyencol North Am 2001;28(3):581–91.
12. Gilstrap LC, Cunningham FG, Whalley PJ. Acute pyelonephritis in pregnancy: an anterospective study. Obstet Gynecol 1981;57:409–13.
13. Cunningham FG. Urinary tract infections complicating pregnancy. Clin Obstet Gynecol 1987;1:891–908.
14. Cunningham G, Lucas M. Urinary tract infections complicating pregnancy. Ballieres Clin Obstet Gynecol 1994;8(2):353–73.
15. American Academy of Pediatrics and American College of Obstetricians and Gynecologists. Guidelines for perinatal care. 6th edition. Washington, DC: American Academy of Pediatrics and American College of Obstetricians and Gynecologists; 2007. p. 101.

16. Lin K, Fajardo K. Screening for asymptomatic bacteriuria in adults: evidence for the U.S. Preventive Services Task Force reaffirmation recommendation statement. Ann Intern Med 2008;149:W20–4.
17. Tita A, Andrews WW. Diagnosis and management of clinical chorioamnionitis. Clin Perinatol 2010;37:339–54.
18. Edwards R. Chorioamnionitis and labor. Obstet Gynecol Clin North Am 2005;32: 287–96.
19. Sperling RS, Newton E, Gibbs RS. Intraamniotic infection in low-birth-weight infants. J Infect Dis 1988;157(1):113–7.
20. Waites KB, Katz B, Schelonka RL. Mycoplasmas and ureaplasmas as neonatal pathogens. Clin Microbiol Rev 2005;18(4):757–89.
21. Gibbs RS, Dinsmoor MJ, Newton ER, et al. A randomized trial of intrapartum versus postpartum treatment of women with intraamniotic infection. Obstet Gynecol 1988;72:823–8.
22. Gilstrap LC, Leveno KJ, Cox SM, et al. Intrapartum treatment of acute chorioamnionitis: impact on neonatal sepsis. Am J Obstet Gynecol 1988;159(3):579–83.
23. Newton ER. Chorioamnionitis and intraamniotic infection. Clin Obstet Gynecol 1993;36:795–808.
24. Sawaya GF, Grady D, Kerlikowske K, et al. Antibiotics at the time of induced abortion: the case for universal prophylaxis based on a meta-analysis. Obstet Gynecol 1996;87:884–90.
25. Fjerstad M, Trussell J, Sivin I, et al. Rates of serious infection after changes in regimens for medical abortion. N Engl J Med 2009;361:145–51.
26. Rios FG, Risso-Vazquez A, Alvarez J, et al. Clinical characteristics and outcomes of obstetric patients admitted to the intensive care unit. Int J Gynaecol Obstet 2012;119:136–40.
27. Berg CJ, Callaghan WM, Syverson C, et al. Pregnancy-related mortality in the United States, 1998-2005. Obstet Gynecol 2010;116:1302–9.
28. Khan KS, Wodjyla D, Say, et al. WHO analysis of causes of maternal death: a systematic review. Lancet 2006;367:1066–74.
29. Stubblefield PG, Grimes DA. Septic abortion. N Engl J Med 1994;33:310–4.
30. Aldape MJ, Bryant AE, Stevens DL. *Clostridium sordellii* infection: epidemiology, clinical findings and current perspectives on diagnosis and treatment. Clin Infect Dis 2006;43:1436–46.
31. Zane S, Guarner J. Gynecologic clostridial toxic shock in women of reproductive age. Curr Infect Dis Rep 2011;13:561–70.
32. Faro S. Postpartum endometritis. Clin Perinatol 2005;32:803–14.
33. Gilstrap LC, Cunningham FG. The bacterial pathogenesis of infection following cesarean section. Obstet Gynecol 1979;53:545–9.
34. Filker RS, Monif GR. Postpartum septicemia due to group G streptococci. Obstet Gynecol 1979;53(Suppl 3):28S–30S.
35. French LM, Smaill FM. Antibiotic regimens for endometritis after delivery. Cochrane Database Syst Rev 2002;(1):CD001067.
36. Brumfield CG, Hauth JC, Andrews WW. Puerperal infection after cesarean delivery: evaluation of a standardized protocol. Am J Obstet Gynecol 2000; 182:1147.
37. Brown CEL, Stettler RW, Twickler D, et al. Puerperal septic pelvic thrombophlebitis: incidence and response to heparin therapy. Am J Obstet Gynecol 1999;181:183.
38. American College of Obstetrics and Gynecology. Use of prophylactic antibiotics in labor and delivery. Practice Bulletin 120. Washington, DC: American College of Obstetrics and Gynecology; 2011.

39. Klevens RM, Edwards JR, Richards CL Jr, et al. Estimating health care-associated infections and deaths in U.S. hospitals, 2002. Public Health Rep 2007;122:160–6.
40. Centers for Disease Control and Prevention. Guideline for prevention of surgical site infection. Infect Control Hosp Epidemiol 1999;20(4):247–78.
41. Faro C, Faro S. Postoperative pelvic infections. Infect Dis Clin North Am 2008;22: 653–63.
42. Larsen JW, Hager WD, Livengood CH, et al. Guidelines for the diagnosis, treatment and prevention of postoperative infections. Infect Dis Obstet Gynecol 2003;11:65–70.
43. Demey HE, Hautekeete ML, Buytaert P, et al. Mastitis and toxic shock syndrome. Acta Obstet Gynecol Scand 1989;68(1):87–8.
44. Fujiwara Y, Endo S. A case of toxic shock syndrome secondary to mastitis caused by methicillin-resistant *Staphylococcus aureus*. Kansenshogaku Zasshi 2001; 75(10):898–903 [in Japanese].
45. Laibl VR, Sheffield JS, Roberts SW, et al. Clinical presentation of community-acquired methicillin-resistant *Staphylococcus aureus* in pregnancy. Obstet Gynecol 2005;106(3):461–5.
46. Stafford I, Hernandez J, Laibl V, et al. Community-acquired methicillin-resistant *Staphylococcus aureus* among patients with puerperal mastitis requiring hospitalization. Obstet Gynecol 2008;112(3):533–7.
47. Oxorn H. The changing aspects of pneumonia complicating pregnancy. Am J Obstet Gynecol 1955;70(5):1057–63.
48. Jin Y, Carrlere KC, Marrie TJ, et al. The effects of community-acquired pneumonia during pregnancy ending with a live birth. Am J Obstet Gynecol 2003;188:800–6.
49. Yost NP, Bloom SL, Richey SD, et al. An appraisal of treatment guidelines for antepartum community-acquired pneumonia. Am J Obstet Gynecol 2000;183(1): 131–5.
50. Chen YH, Keller J, Wang IT, et al. Pneumonia and pregnancy outcomes: a nationwide population-based study. Am J Obstet Gynecol 2012;207:288.e1–7.
51. Mandell LA, Wunderink RG, Anqueto A, et al. Infectious Disease Society of American/American Thoracic Society consensus guidelines on the management of community-acquired pneumonia in adults. Clin Infect Dis 2007;44(Suppl 2): S27–72.
52. Rotas M, McCalla S, Liu C, et al. Methicillin-resistant *Staphylococcus aureus* necrotizing pneumonia arising from an infected episiotomy site. Obstet Gynecol 2007;109:533–6.
53. Durrington HJ, Summers C. Recent changes in the management of community-acquired pneumonia in adults. BMJ 2008;336:1429–33.
54. Nuzum JW, Pilot I, Stangl FH, et al. Pandemic influenza and pneumonia in a large civilian hospital. JAMA 1918;71(19):1562–5.
55. Mazze RI, Källén B. Appendectomy during pregnancy: a Swedish registry study of 778 cases. Obstet Gynecol 1991;77:835.
56. Gearhart SL, Silen W. Acute appendicitis and peritonitis. In: Fauci AS, Braunwald E, Kasper DL, et al, editors. Harrison's principles of internal medicine. 17th edition. New York: McGraw-Hill; 2008. p. 1914.
57. Hodjati H, Kazerooni T. Location of the appendix in the gravid patient: a re-evaluation of the established concept. Int J Gynaecol Obstet 2003;81:245–7.
58. Valdivieso V, Covarrubias C, Siegel F, et al. Pregnancy and cholelithiasis: pathogenesis and natural course of gallstones diagnosed in early puerperium. Hepatology 1993;17:1

59. Glasgow RE, Visser BC, Harris HW, et al. Changing management of gallstone disease during pregnancy. Surg Endosc 1998;12:241.
60. Barone JE, Bears S, Chen S, et al. Outcome study of cholecystectomy during pregnancy. Am J Surg 1999;177:232.
61. Mazurek GH, Jereb J, Lobue P, et al, Centers for Disease Control and Prevention. Guidelines for using the Quantiferon-TB Gold Test for detecting *Mycobacterium tuberculosis* infection, United States. MMWR Recomm Rep 2005;54(RR–12): 49–55.
62. Brost BC, Newman KB. The maternal effects of tuberculosis therapy. Obstet Gynecol Clin North Am 1997;24:659.
63. Centers for Disease Control and Prevention. Treatment of tuberculosis. MMWR Recomm Rep 2003;52(RR–11):1–77.
64. Fernandez-Perez ER, Salman S, Pendem S, et al. Sepsis during pregnancy. Crit Care Med 2005;33:S286–93.
65. Neligan PJ, Laffey JF. Clinical review: special populations-critical illness and pregnancy. Crit Care 2011;15:227.
66. Jenkins TM, Troiano NH, Graves CR, et al. Mechanical ventilation in an obstetric population: characteristics and delivery rates. Am J Obstet Gynecol 2003;188(2): 549–52.
67. Clark SL, Cotton DB, Lee W, et al. Central hemodynamic assessment of normal term pregnancy. Am J Obstet Gynecol 1989;161:1439–42.
68. Bakker J, Gris P, Coffernils M, et al. Serial blood lactate levels can predict the development of multiple organ failure following septic shock. Am J Surg 1996; 171:221–6.
69. Benedetti TJ, Carlson RW. Studies of colloid osmotic pressure in pregnancy-induced hypertension. Am J Obstet Gynecol 1979;135:308.
70. Mendenhall HW. Serum protein concentrations in pregnancy. 1. Conentrations in maternal serum. Am J Obstet Gynecol 1970;106:388.
71. Rivers E, Nguyen B, Havstad S, et al. Early goal-directed therapy in the treatment of severe sepsis and septic shock. N Engl J Med 2001;345:1368–77.
72. Abdel-Wahab OI, Healy B, Dzik WH. Effect of fresh-frozen plasma transfusion on pro-thrombin time and bleeding in patients with mild coagulation abnormalities. Transfusion 2006;46:1279–85.
73. College of American Pathologists. Practice parameter for the use of fresh-frozen plasma, cryoprecipitate, and platelets. JAMA 1994;271:777–81.
74. American Society of Anaesthesiologists. Task Force on Blood Component Therapy: practice guidelines for blood component therapy. Anesthesiology 1996;84:732–47.
75. Ferrer R, Artigas A, Levy MM, et al. Improvement in process of care an outcome after a multicenter severe sepsis educational program in Spain. JAMA 2008;299: 2294–303.
76. Robson WP, Daniels R. The sepsis six: helping patients to survive sepsis. Br J Nurs 2008;17:16–21.
77. Robson W, Nutbeam T, Daniels R. Sepsis and need for pre-hospital intervention? Emerg Med J 2009;26:535–8.
78. Daniels R, Nutbeam I, McNamara G, et al. The sepsis six and severe sepsis resuscitation bundle: a prospective observational cohort study. Emerg Med J 2011 Jun;28(6):507–12.
79. Dellinger RP, Levy MM, Carlet JM, et al. Surviving Sepsis Campaign: international guidelines for management of severe sepsis and septic shock: 2008. Crit Care Med 2008;36:296–327.

Hypertensive Emergencies of Pregnancy

James M. Alexander, MD*, Karen L. Wilson, MD

KEYWORDS

- Hypertensive emergency • Preeclampsia • Antihypertensive medication • Stroke
- Blood pressure

KEY POINTS

- Hypertensive crisis is a severe complication that can result in catastrophic consequences.
- Immediate stabilization of the mother including the use of intravenous antihypertensives is required and delivery is often indicated.
- Fetal well-being should be confirmed through fetal monitoring and ultrasound.
- There are several antihypertensive agents that are appropriate and safe for use in pregnancy.

Hypertension is commonly encountered in pregnancy, impacting 10% of all gestations.[1] Although sometimes caused by preexisting chronic hypertension and related to other comorbidities, more commonly hypertension encountered during pregnancy develops spontaneously. When this happens beyond 20 weeks of gestation and returns to normal levels postpartum, the National High Blood Pressure Education Program Working Group recommends that the term gestational hypertension be used. This group has categorized hypertensive disease of pregnancy into the following 5 groups (**Table 1**)[2]:

- Gestational hypertension—Previously this was termed pregnancy-induced hypertension. If preeclampsia does not develop and the elevated blood pressure (BP) resolves postpartum, it is termed transient hypertension.
- Preeclampsia—Diagnosed when the BP is elevated and proteinuria is present.
- Eclampsia—Tonic-clonic seizures due to preeclampsia or gestational hypertension.
- Chronic hypertension with superimposed preeclampsia—Underlying hypertension with the development of preeclampsia during pregnancy.
- Chronic hypertension—Hypertension that is present at the time of conception.

Department of Obstetrics and Gynecology, University of Texas Southwestern Medical Center, 5323 Harry Hines Boulevard, Dallas, TX 75390-9032, USA
* Corresponding author.
E-mail address: James.Alexander@UTsouthwestern.edu

Obstet Gynecol Clin N Am 40 (2013) 89–101
http://dx.doi.org/10.1016/j.ogc.2012.11.008
0889-8545/13/$ – see front matter © 2013 Elsevier Inc. All rights reserved.

Table 1
National High Blood Pressure Education Program's Working Group Classification

Category	Definition
Gestational hypertension	• Hypertension develops during the pregnancy • No proteinuria • If the hypertension resolves by the 12th postpartum week, the diagnosis is changed to transient hypertension
Chronic hypertension	• Hypertension present before pregnancy or diagnosed before the 20th wk of gestation • Hypertension that is diagnosed during the pregnancy and fails to resolve by 12 wk postpartum is retrospectively diagnosed as chronic hypertension

Chronic hypertension with superimposed preeclampsia	• Underlying diagnosis of hypertension
	• Development of
	  ○ Worsening hypertension after 20 wk
	  ○ New onset of proteinuria
	  ○ Development of other signs and symptoms of preeclampsia

Preeclampsia	• New onset hypertension
	• More than 300 mg protein in a 24-h urine collection
	• The diagnosis is more certain if any one of the following is present
	  ○ Blood pressure >160 mm Hg or >110 mm Hg
	  ○ Proteinuria >2 g/24 h or 2+ by dipstick
	  ○ Severe creatinine level >1.2 mg/dL
	  ○ Platelet count <100,000 cells/mm^3
	  ○ Elevated liver enzymes
	  ○ Persistent headache or other cerebral or visual disturbances
	  ○ Persistent epigastric pain

Eclampsia	• Tonic clonic seizure • Any of the above hypertensive scenarios

Data from National High Blood Pressure Education Program: Working Group Report on High Blood Pressure in Pregnancy. Am J Obstet Gynecol 2000;183:S1–S22.

According to the criteria developed by this group, gestational hypertension requires a BP of 140/90 to establish the diagnosis; as many as one-quarter of these will go on to develop proteinuria (ie, preeclampsia).[3] Preeclampsia is the syndrome defined as an elevation of the BP with new-onset proteinuria and in more serious cases may include signs or symptoms of multiorgan involvement. These additional associated signs and symptoms indicate more serious pathophysiology and, if the criteria in **Table 2** are met, is referred to as severe preeclampsia.

Historically, hypertension has been one of the more common causes of mortality in pregnancy. As recently as the 1930s, the maternal rate of mortality was 1% in the Western world and hypertension accounted for 20% of these deaths.[4] Said another way, 2 of every 1000 women died because of a hypertensive-related diagnosis during pregnancy. Although maternal rate of mortality is greatly decreased now with recent data showing an incidence of 15/100,000 in the United States, the proportion of deaths due to hypertension remains high at 10% or more (**Table 3**).[5,6] Untoward pregnancy outcomes encompass both the mother and the fetus with the fetus suffering increased mortality as well, both from direct impacts of hypertension, which

Table 2
Criteria for severe preeclampsia

Signs or Symptom of Preeclampsia	Severe (Present)	Mild (Absent)
Blood pressure ≥160/110	Yes	No
Liver enzyme elevation	Yes	No
Thrombocytopenia (platelets <100,000/mm³)	Yes	No
Elevated creatinine (≥1.2 mg/dL)	Yes	No
Persistent headache or visual disturbances	Yes	No
Proteinuria ≥2 g in a 24-h period[a]	Yes	No
Oliguria	Yes	No
Oligohydramnios or fetal growth restriction	Yes	No

[a] Thresholds vary depending on source.

include oligohydramnios, growth restriction, and stillbirth, and from the impact of delivering prematurely.[7,8] There is no cure for gestational hypertension, and the disorder only goes away after termination of the pregnancy. Too often this is necessary early in the third trimester, resulting in a preterm infant that does not always survive or suffers severe morbidity because of the complications of prematurity.

This article focuses on a specific group of pregnancies complicated by very elevated BPs, those that experience hypertensive crisis or emergencies. Typically this occurs in women with severe preeclampsia, but it can also occur in women with uncontrolled chronic hypertension before 20 weeks. The prognosis for a successful outcome in this latter group of women is understandably poor and these pregnancies are often complicated by comorbidities such as diabetes or other chronic disease. In addition to discussion about the maternal and fetal consequences of a hypertensive emergency, evaluation and treatment are considered with guidelines for the clinician provided.

Table 3
Causes of maternal death

	Berg N = 108 (%)	Clark N = 95 (%)
Pregnancy-related		
Hypertension	10 (9)	15 (16)
Cardiomyopathy	21 (19)	10 (11)
Hemorrhage	14 (13)	11 (12)
Infection	7 (6)	7 (7)
Embolism	13 (12)	22 (23)
Non–pregnancy-related		
Cardiovascular condition	5 (5)	–
Chronic illness	9 (8)	–
Nonobstetric infection	–	7 (7)
Accident	–	6 (6)
Miscellaneous/other	29 (27)	17 (18)

Data from Berg CJ, Chang J, Callaghan WM, et al. Pregnancy-related mortality in the United States 1991–1997. Obstet Gynecol 2003;101:289; and Clark SL, Belfort MA, Dildy GA, et al. Maternal death in the 21st century: causes, prevention, and relationship to cesarean delivery. Am J Obstet Gynecol 2008;199(1):36.e1.

CONSEQUENCES OF A HYPERTENSIVE EMERGENCY

The maternal consequences of severe hypertension are many and are related to end-organ damage. In pregnancy this is primarily manifested in the kidney, brain, uterus, and lungs. Fortunately the individual has a remarkable ability to maintain organ perfusion with varying degrees of BP by autoregulatory mechanisms. It is only after these mechanisms reach their limit that end-organ dysfunction and tissue damage occur. In nonpregnant individuals, a hypertensive crisis is often described as a systolic BP ≥180 or a diastolic BP ≥120 with further characterization as hypertensive urgency or emergency based on the degree and acuteness of the elevation.[9–12] The BP threshold in pregnancy is generally a bit lower due to the pathophysiology, maternal age, and recognition that the consequences can be severe with severe morbidity to both the mother and the fetus.[3]

Cardiovascular

Preeclampsia impacts cardiovascular function during pregnancy in several ways:

- Increased afterload: in normal pregnancy vasodilation and a decrease in afterload typically exists. Hypertension reverses this state as increasing systemic vascular resistance.
- Decreased preload: this is variable and caused by decreased volume expansion that sometimes occurs in women who develop preeclampsia: pregnancy is typically associated with a 50% increase in blood volume. However, this expansion is diminished and even absent in preeclamptic women.
- Endothelial injury with extravasation of intravascular fluid into the extracellular space, especially the lungs.

Several studies of preeclamptic and eclamptic women using invasive hemodynamic methods have evaluated the cardiac function of these women and the factors that impact cardiac output. Several studies have demonstrated that the reduction in cardiac output at the onset of preeclampsia is due to increased peripheral resistance.[13–16] Hankins and colleagues[14] demonstrated that these women are in a hyperdynamic state. Although the women are in a hyperdynamic state, filling pressures in the left ventricle were primarily dependent on intravenous fluid administration, with aggressive fluids increasing left ventricular stroke work. This hyperdynamic state was accompanied by increased pulmonary capillary wedge pressure and was associated with pulmonary edema.[15,16] In hypertensive crisis and the resultant elevation in afterload, the decrease in cardiac output is even greater and the risk of pulmonary edema higher.

Renal

In normal pregnancy, increased blood volume and renal blood flow result in a dramatic increase in glomerular filtration rate (GFR) and creatine clearance.[17,18] Preeclamptic women often have a decreased volume expansion of pregnancy that impacts renal flow and the GFR filtration rate.[19,20] In addition, renal artery vasospasm can lead to a significant enough decrease in the GFR that oliguria results.[21] This oliguria can be quite pronounced in the most severe cases and urine output can decrease to as low as 10 to 20 milliliters per hour. Vigorous intravenous resuscitation with crystalloid may increase urine output by a modest amount; however, there is a very real risk of pulmonary edema with vigorous hydration due to increased pulmonary capillary wedge pressure and endothelial leak. In the absence of acute hemorrhage, aggressive hydration should be avoided.

The endothelial damage seen in preeclampsia leads to dysfunction of the glomerular apparatus of the kidney.[22–24] Glomeruli are enlarged; endothelial cells are swollen, and subendothelial deposits of proteins and fibrins have been seen using electron microscopy. These changes are associated with significant leakage of protein into the urine such that it may approach nephrotic range.

Uterine

Before the development of the clinical manifestations of preeclampsia, changes are evident in the placenta; the result is compromised uterine blood flow. In normal pregnancy, the spiral arteries undergo extensive remolding as they are invaded by the trophoblast. This remodeling is incomplete in preeclamptic women, leading to abnormal trophoblastic invasion and spiral arteries that are narrower, resulting impaired placental blood flow.[25–27] This compromised placental blood flow is sometimes manifested by abnormal fetal growth, oligohydramnios, and even stillbirth. The risk of abruption is elevated as well. In hypertensive crisis, acute disruption of uterine artery flow to the placenta can occur, leading to sudden fetal decompensation. Continuous electronic fetal monitoring, a sonogram for fetal growth, and amniotic fluid assessment are recommended for these women.

Neurologic

The most recognized and obvious neurologic complication of preeclampsia is eclampsia. It is characterized as a violent, tonic-clonic seizure that can be recurrent if untreated and will eventually lead to a comatose state and death. In addition to eclampsia, stroke is a feared complication of severe preeclampsia and is seen in acutely hypertensive patients when the systemic BP exceeds 160/110 mm Hg. Older studies of women who died from hypertension in pregnancy demonstrate that greater than half of eclamptics suffer intracranial hemorrhage, although this was the cause of death in less than half of the women.[28–30] Other pathologic abnormalities seen included cortical and subcortical hemorrhages including the occipital lobe, numerous small cortical infarctions, and subcortical edema. More rarely, magnetic resonance imaging (MRI) has been used to characterize the brain lesions seen in preeclamptic women exhibiting neurologic manifestations. In addition to the anatomic findings described above, posterior reversible encephalopathy syndrome (PRES) has been described.[31–34]

PRES is a disorder seen in the setting of acute elevation of BP in both pregnant and nonpregnant individuals and is a result of the failure of cerebral autoregulation of cerebral blood flow (CBF). Cerebral autoregulation maintains a constant CBF in the face of hypertension through vasoconstriction of the afferent arterioles.[35,36] Through this mechanism, capillary damage and cerebral edema are avoided; however, this mechanism is only able to maintain CBF across a certain range. With a systemic BP of >160/110, cerebral autoregulation begins to fail and brain injury can occur. Increased CBF produces hyperperfusion, disruption of the blood-brain barrier, and edema formation.[37] PRES presents with headaches, nausea, altered mental function, visual disturbances, and seizure. On MRI, a characteristic appearance is seen with T2 hypersensitivity on fluid attenuation inversion recovery images showing vasogenic edema, especially in the occipital lobe and sometimes subcortical infarctions.[34] These changes typically resolve postpartum, although there is now evidence that some are persistent and present several weeks after delivery.[34,38,39] The long-term significance of these persistent lesions is not well studied or understood.

Cerebral hemorrhage and stroke can occur with severely elevated BP and is one of the most devastating complications of preeclampsia because of the permanent and irreversible damage that occurs. Sudden death associated with massive cerebral hemorrhage can also occur and is more likely in older women with longstanding hypertension. More commonly, hemorrhage occurs in areas of cerebral ischemia and infarction. Subarachnoid hemorrhage can also occur and blood can be seen over the convexity of the frontal/partial lobes and into the sylvian tissue and interhemispheric tissue. Computed tomographic scanning should not be used to identify PRES (MRI is the modality of choice); however, computed tomographic scanning is excellent at identifying intracranial hemorrhage and is more readily available in the acute setting. In women presenting with acute hypertensive crisis and any lateralizing findings on neurologic examination, consideration should be given for immediate neuroimaging, often a computed tomographic scan.

Visual disturbances that occur with preeclampsia and severe BP elevation include scotomata, amaurosis, and blurred vision.[40,41] These visual disturbances are usually due to the involvement of the cortical lobe in the neurologic changes previously described, but may also be due to retinal abnormalities including detachment. These visual changes are typically reversible with BP control and delivery of the fetus.

PHARMACOLOGIC THERAPY
General Considerations

The goal of therapy in a woman experiencing severe elevation of her BP is to lower the pressure to a level that minimizes end-organ damage while avoiding hypotension.[2] Overly aggressive treatment that leads to hypotension can impact uterine perfusion, resulting in fetal distress. Fetal distress can sometimes be seen in the fetal heart rate tracing, which may show decelerations, loss of beat-to-beat variability, and even bradycardia. Depending on the agent used, the mother may experience rebound tachycardia, headache, palpitations, flushing, anxiety, tremors, and vomiting. Careful attention must be given to not only the choice of drug but also the appropriate dosing, including the amount and interval. Faced with an acute hypertensive event, the practitioner feels the need to bring the BP down to safe levels very quickly, which can lead to inappropriate and too frequent dosing of the medication.

Patients with hypertensive crisis require hospitalization and treatment in an acute care setting. These patients are quite ill and can suddenly decompensate. Although administering antihypertensive medication, monitoring the mother and fetus, including frequent checking of maternal pulse and BP as well as continuous fetal monitoring, is required until the BP is in a safe range. Extreme BP elevation that results in a systolic BP >200 or a diastolic BP >120 usually requires intensive care unit admission. These women are at particular risk of an acute myocardial infarction, encephalopathy, stroke, dissecting aneurysm, acute renal failure, and pulmonary edema second to left ventricular failure.[9–12]

Specific Agents Used for Treating Hypertensive Crisis

There is no consensus as to what pharmacologic therapy is ideal for the treatment of acute hypertensive crisis in pregnancy. Aldomet is one of the longest used and has one of the safest medication profiles in pregnancy. Although Aldomet can be effective in treating chronic hypertension in pregnancy, it is ineffective in hypertensive crisis. Angiotensin-converting enzyme inhibitors are often used first line in nonpregnant patients with heart failure, pulmonary edema, or acute coronary ischemia but this class of drugs is contraindicated in pregnancy because of the risk of renal dysgenesis, oligohydramnios, and fetal growth restriction.[41] In those cases of hypertensive crisis that occur postpartum, angiotensin converting enzyme inhibitors can be quite useful

Diuretics

Diuretics are not commonly used unless the hypertensive crisis is associated with pulmonary edema or congestive heart failure. Even then, their use in the setting of severe preeclampsia is problematic because these patients are intravascular depleted due to inadequate pregnancy-related volume expansion and endothelial leak. A vigorous diuresis can further constrict the intravascular space and lead to further underperfusion of end organs. The uterus is of particular concern because the fetus may not tolerate the underperfusion, especially when growth restriction is present. In the absence of pulmonary edema or congestive heart failure, diuretic use is most commonly seen postpartum to help facilitate the diuretics commonly seen in the preeclamptic patient.[20,42]

Hydralazine

Hydralazine, administered intravenously, has been the most commonly used drug in pregnancy for the last 50 years. It is a peripheral vasodilator that impacts maternal and fetal placental circulation. Hydralazine is thought to reduce peripheral vascular resistance and systemic BP through the relaxation of precapillary arterioles. The onset of effect is within 10 to 20 minutes and dosing should occur at 15- to 20-minute intervals until the desired BP effect is achieved. It is recommended that an initial dose of 5 mg be given followed by 10-mg doses as needed.[3] This recommendation is because a small number of women will have a very pronounced response and become hypotensive. The effect of hydralazine therapy is not limited to maternal hemodynamics. Jouppila and colleagues[43] demonstrated that umbilical vein flow was increased irrespective of maternal heart rate, BP, or intervillous blood flow, suggesting that vasodilation occurs in the umbilical vessels. Harper and Murnaghan also demonstrated improved placental circulation, likely because of vasodilation.[44]

Side effects are common and affect up to 50% of treated patients. They include reflex tachycardia, hypotensive headache, palpitations, flushing, anxiety, tremors, vomiting, epigastric pain, and fluid retention. In general, these effects are short lived and not dangerous; however, in a small number of patients, overshoot hypotension can occur, especially in intravascularly volume-depleted patients. The fetal response to maternal hypertension and the subsequent placenta hypoperfusion is often fetal heart rate declinations and even bradycardia. Maternal position changes and intravenous fluids will usually improve this situation. The 5-mg dose mentioned above and an appropriate dosing internal can minimize the risk of hypertension.

β-blocker

Intravenous labetalol has been used increasingly for hypertensive crisis. It is a selective α1 and nonselective β-blocker with more of a β effect than an α effect. Labetalol decreases systemic vascular resistance and decreases the HR peripheral and decreased peripheral vascular resistance and BP. It does this without reducing peripheral blood flow and preserves cerebral, renal, and coronary circulation. Likewise, uteroplacental flow is unchanged. Labetalol is typically given in intravenous boluses, starting with 20 mg and repeating every 20 minutes as needed. If the 20-mg dose is ineffective, 40, 60, or even 80 mg can be given with the doses being escalated until the desired effect is achieved.[2,3,45] The onset of action of labetalol is relatively quick, within 5 minutes, and its effect can last up to 6 hours.

Although usually well tolerated, labetalol, like hydralazine, can cause overshoot hypertension with a subsequent fetal effect. This, however, seems less frequent than with hydralazine and does not cause maternal rebound tachycardia. The lack of rebound tachycardia and the small risk of hypotension make labetalol a particularly good choice in patients with congestive heart failure or in those who have experienced myocardial infarction. It should not be administered with a calcium channel blocker because of the risk of cardiac depression. Esmolol is the very short-acting intravenous β-blocker that has seen limited use in pregnancy. Ducey and Knap have reported an unacceptable risk of cesarean delivery for fetal distress with its use.[46]

Calcium channel blockers

Nifedipine is an oral calcium channel blocker used primarily for tocolysis, but has seen increased use for hypertension in pregnancy. Ten-milligram capsules can be given orally for acute control of hypertension for up to 3 doses.[2,47] It has been reported to have as rapid an onset as intravenous labetalol and to be just as effective. Unlike labetalol, nifedipine acts as a renal artery vasodilator and natriuretic, resulting in increased urine output. It also increases the cardiac index and lowers BP without impacting uterine placental blood flow and without fetal heart rate abnormalities. Like hydralazine and labetalol, unexpected hypertension can result in full distress.

Unexpected and unpredictable decreases in BP have occurred with nifedipine capsules, resulting in the withdrawal of short-acting nifedipine for the market in Australia and some US pharmacies.[48] Interaction between $MgSO_4$ and calcium channel blocker is of some concern and case reports have shown severe hypotension, neuromuscular blockage, and symptomatic hypotension.[49] A case control study of 162 cases who received MgSO and nifedipine concluded that nifedipine and magnesium together do not increase adverse effects or hypotension. The Magpie trial reported on 3029 women who received both nifedipine and magnesium.[50] A similar incidence of hypertension was seen in the women receiving nifedipine and magnesium (0.4%) and those receiving nifedipine and placebo (0.3%). Rahen and colleagues report similar results.

Nitroprusside

Nitroprusside has been used sporadically in pregnancy but only in the most severe cases of hypertension.[2] Complications due to excessive vasodilation in volume-depleted preeclamptic women have been reported.[51] Cardiac output can actually decrease with its administration because of the resultant decrease in preload as a result of hypotension. Another concern about its use in pregnancy is related to the production of cyanide during its metabolism.[52] The risk of fetal cyanide toxicity as a result is unknown. Due to the long experience with hydralazine and the more recent successful experience with labetalol and calcium channel blockers, the use of nitroprusside should be limited to those cases refractory to other therapy.

COMPARISON OF DOSING REGIMENS

There have been several comparison studies of the most commonly used drugs for acute control of hypertension. Several of these have compared intravenous hydralazine to labetalol. A recent metaanalysis[53,54] provides a nice summary of these trials. Although the analysis showed hydralazine equally effective as labetalol, it was less effective than nifedipine and associated with poorer maternal and perinatal outcomes. The authors concluded that hydralazine should not be used as a first-line agent. This analysis should be interpreted with caution, however, because several small and quasirandomized trials were included and the confidence intervals around the outcomes were very high. Urban and colleagues[55] came to a different conclusion and suggested that objective data did not support the use of one agent over another. Vigil-de Gracia and colleagues[56] randomized 200 severely hypertensive patients to labetalol versus labetalol given in escalating doses. Maternal and neonatal outcomes were similar with more maternal tachycardia seen with hydralazine use and more hypoplasia and bradycardia were seen with labetalol use.

Studies comparing labetalol to nifedipine have also been conducted. Rahen and colleagues randomized 50 women to either oral nifedipine given in 10-mg doses or intravenous labetalol given in an escalating dose regime of 20, 40, and 80 mg. The 2 regimens were shown to be rapidly effective without significant adverse effect on either maternal or infant outcomes. These findings were similar in many respects to an earlier trial conducted by Vermillion and colleagues.[52] Like Rahen, Vermillion and coworkers concluded that nifedipine and labetalol were equally effective in the management of acute hypertensive emergencies; however, they found that nifedipine controlled hypertension more rapidly and caused a significant increase in urinary output.[52] In a separate article generated from the same study, Scardo and colleagues[57] also reported an increase in the cardiac index with nifedipine. A recent Cochrane review of hydralazine, labetalol, and nifedipine concluded that, until better evidence is available, the choice of antihypertensive should depend on the clinician's experience, familiarity with a particular drug, and what is known about adverse effects.[58]

EVALUATION AND TREATMENT

The first step in the evaluation of the patient who presents with a hypertensive crisis is to determine the BP accurately. The patient should be hospitalized and the physician should then determine if signs or symptoms of end-organ damage are present, focusing on neurologic, cardiac, renal, and fetal signs (including maternal perception of activity) of decompensation. A thorough examination and evaluation should be performed (**Box 1**). Most cases of severe hypertension are diagnosed in the setting of preeclampsia and the initial evaluation is focused with this in mind. Immediate

---

Box 1
Evaluation of the pregnancy complicated by hypertensive crisis

Stabilization

- Admission to the hospital
- Blood pressure assessment every 15 to 30 minutes
- Administration of intravenous antihypertensive agents

Assessment of fetal well-being

- Electronic fetal heart rate monitoring
- Ultrasound for fetal growth and amniotic fluid assessment

Determination of cause

- Review of history focusing on identification of underlying comorbidities, including chronic hypertension, renal disease, and diabetes
- Evaluation of the presence of preeclampsia

Assessment of secondary complication

- Neuroimaging to identify intracranial hemorrhage if the neurologic examination is abnormal
- Cardiopulmonary monitoring, which may include echocardiography, echocardiography, and/or chest radiography
- Serum creatinine to assess renal function

laboratory evaluation should include serum creatinine, levels of liver transaminase, and a hemogram to include platelets. Many of these patients will have comorbidities and assessment of these should occur as indicated. This assessment may include an echocardiogram.

The fetus is at risk of acute decompensation during hypertensive crisis and should be evaluated quickly. Signs of fetal compromise include abnormal growth, decreased amniotic fluid, and abnormal fetal heart rate tracing. An initial sonogram to determine an estimated fetal weight and amniotic fluid index should be performed and continuous fetal monitoring should be initiated. Because the therapy to decrease the BP can adversely impact uterine perfusion, electronic fetal monitoring should continue until the crisis is resolved.

Attempts to decrease the BP should occur quickly using one of the regimens described above. Although there is no ideal regimen that can currently be recommended, several caveats of therapies are in order. First, any regimen used should be familiar to the physician and the proper dosing schedule should be adhered to as single-agent therapy. Second, treatment of actual elevated BP is primarily for the benefit of the mother and can in fact further compromise the fetus if one is overly aggressive. von Dadelszen and colleagues[59,60] have documented a correlation between a decrease in mean arterial pressure and fetal growth restriction. Magee and colleagues[54] were unable to demonstrate any reduction in fetal growth restriction, abruption, or improved prenatal outcomes with acute BP control. Third, if the underlying case is preeclampsia, consideration for delivery should be given.

Occasionally, hypertensive crisis will be seen early in pregnancy related to uncontrolled chronic hypertension. Once acute control is established, long-term control with oral therapy is pursued.

SUMMARY

Hypertensive crisis is a serious condition that is sometimes encountered in pregnancy, especially in women who are preeclamptic. The consequences can be catastrophic and include seizures, cerebrovascular accident, cardiopulmonary decompensation and failure, renal compromise, fetal distress, and stillbirth. Women with BPs >160/110 must be quickly identified and treatment initiated rapidly to prevent adverse outcomes. There are several choices of antihypotensive agents available to the clinicians that are appropriate and safe to administer in pregnancy. These antihypotensive agents include hydralazine, labetalol, and calcium channel blockers. Although there are pros and cons to the choice of any of these agents, the clinician should use the drug the clinicians are most familiar with and that is most readily available to them in the labor and delivery unit. Attention should be given to the fetus and the fetus' well-being should be confirmed with fetal monitoring and ultrasonography as indicated. After initial assessment and stabilization occur, the determination of the cause of the hypertensive crisis should be pursued. Often this will be preeclampsia and, in many cases, delivery of the fetus will be required. Identification of the women at risk, acute intervention, and treatment of the underlying cause of the elevation of BP will lead to excellent maternal and fetal outcomes in most cases.

REFERENCES

1. Martin JA, Hamilton BE, Sutton PD, et al. Births: final data for 2004. Natl Vital Stat Rep 2006;55:1–101.
2. National High Blood Pressure Education Program: Working Group Report on High Blood Pressure in Pregnancy. Am J Obstet Gynecol 2000;183:51.

3. American College of Obstetricians and Gynecologists: Diagnosis and management of preeclampsia and eclampsia. Practice Bulletin 2002;No. 33.

4. Loudon I. The transformation of maternal mortality. BMJ 1992;305:1557.

5. Clark SL, Belfort MA, Dildy GA, et al. Maternal death in the 21st century: causes, prevention, and relationship to cesarean delivery. Am J Obstet Gynecol 2008; 199(1):36.e1.

6. Berg CJ, Chang J, Callaghan WM, et al. Pregnancy-related mortality in the United States 1991–1997. Obstet Gynecol 2003;101:289.

7. Sibai BM, Barton JR. Expectant management of severe preeclampsia remote from term: patient selection, treatment and delivery indications. Am J Obstet Gynecol 2007;196:514.

8. Sibai BM, Barton JR, Akl S, et al. A randomized prospective comparison of nifedipine and bed rest versus bed rest alone in the management of preeclampsia remote from term. Am J Obstet Gynecol 1992;167(1):879.

9. Papadopoulos DP, Mourouzis I, Thomopoulos C, et al. Hypertension crisis. Blood Press 2010;19:328.

10. Marik P, Varon J. Hypertensive crises, challenges and management. Chest 2007; 131:1949.

11. Deshmukh A, Kumar G, Kumar N, et al. Effect of Joint National Committee VII report on hospitalizations for hypertensive emergencies in the United States. Am J Cardiol 2011;108:1277.

12. Baumann BM, Cline DM, Pimenta E. Treatment of hypertension in the emergency department. J Am Soc Hypertens 2011;5(5):366.

13. Benedetti TJ, Kates R, Williams V. Hemodynamic observations in severe preeclampsia complicated by pulmonary edema. Am J Obstet Gynecol 1985; 152:330.

14. Hankins GD, Wendel GW, Cunningham FG, et al. Longitudinal evaluation of hemodynamic changes in eclampsia. Am J Obstet Gynecol 1984;150:506.

15. Rafferty TD, Berkowitz RL. Hemodynamics in patients with severe toxemia during labor and delivery. Am J Obstet Gynecol 1980;138:263.

16. Phelan JP, Yurth DA. Severe preeclampsia. I. Peripartum hemodynamic observations. Am J Obstet Gynecol 1982;144(1):17.

17. Davison JM, Noble MC. Serial changes in 24-hour creatinine clearance during normal menstrual cycles and the first trimester of pregnancy. Br J Obstet Gynaecol 1981;88:10.

18. Lindheimer MD, Davison JM, Katz AI. The kidney and hypertension in pregnancy: twenty exciting years. Semin Nephrol 2001;21:173.

19. Irons DW, Baylis PH, Butler TJ, et al. Atrial natriuretic peptide in preeclampsia: metabolic clearance, sodium excretion and renal hemodynamics. Am J Physiol 1997;273(3 Pt 2):F483.

20. Zeeman GG, Cunningham FG, Pritchard JA. The magnitude of hemoconcentration with eclampsia. Hypertens Pregnancy 2009;28(2):127–37.

21. Conrad KP, Gaber LW, Lindheimer MD. The kidney in normal pregnancy and preeclampsia. In: Lindheimer MD, Roberts JM, Cunningham FG, editors. Chesley's hypertensive disorders of pregnancy. 3rd edition. New York: Elsevier; 2009. p. 297.

22. Spargo B, McCartney CP, Winemiller R. Glomerular capillary endotheliosis in toxemia of pregnancy. Arch Pathol 1959;68:593.

23. Karumanchi SA, Stillman IE, Lindheimer MD. Angiogenesis and preeclampsia. In: Lindheimer MD, Roberts JM, Cunningham FG, editors. Chesley's hypertensive disorders of pregnancy. 3rd edition. New York: Elsevier; 2009. p. 87.

24. Eremina V, Baelde HJ, Quaggin SE. Role of the VEGF—A signaling pathway in the glomerulus: evidence for crosstalk between components of the glomerular filtration barrier. Nephron Physiol 2007;106(2):32.
25. Hertig AT. Vascular pathology in the hypertensive albuminuric toxemias of pregnancy. Clinics 1945;4:602.
26. Fisher SJ, McMaster M, Roberts JM. The placenta in normal pregnancy and preeclampsia. In: Lindheimer MD, Roberts JM, Cunningham FG, editors. Chesley's hypertensive disorders of pregnancy. 3rd edition. New York: Elsevier; 2009. p. 73.
27. Madazli R, Budak E, Calay Z, et al. Correlation between placental bed biopsy findings, vascular cell adhesion molecule and fibronectin levels in preeclampsia. Br J Obstet Gynaecol 2000;107:514.
28. Melrose EB. Maternal deaths at King Edward VIII Hospital, Durban. A review of 258 consecutive cases. S Afr Med J 1984;65:161.
29. Richards A, Graham DI, Bullock MR. Clinicopathological study of neurological complications due to hypertensive disorders of pregnancy. J Neurol Neurosurg Psychiatry 1988;51:416.
30. Sheehan HL, Lynch JB. Cerebral lesions. In: Pathology of toxaemia of pregnancy. New York: Churchill Livingstone; 1973.
31. Hinchey J, Chaves C, Appignani B, et al. A reversible posterior leukoencephalopathy syndrome. N Engl J Med 1996;334(8):494.
32. Narbone MC, Musolino R, Granata F, et al. PRES: posterior or potentially reversible encephalopathy syndrome? Neurol Sci 2006;27:187.
33. Zeeman GG, Fleckenstein JL, Twickler DM, et al. Cerebral infarction in eclampsia. Am J Obstet Gynecol 2004;190:714.
34. Zeeman GG, Cipolla MJ, Cunningham FG. Cerebrovascular pathophysiology in preeclampsia/eclampsia. In: Lindheimer MD, Roberts JM, Cunningham FG, editors. Chesley's hypertensive disorders in pregnancy. 3rd edition. New York: Elsevier; 2009. p. 227.
35. Cipolla MJ, Smith J, Kohlmeyer MM, et al. SKCa and IKCa channels, myogenic tone, and vasodilator responses in middle cerebral arteries and parenchymal arterioles: effect of ischemia and reperfusion. Stroke 2009;40(4):1451.
36. Cipolla MJ. Brief review: cerebrovascular function during pregnancy and eclampsia. Hypertension 2007;50:14.
37. Cunningham FG, Twickler D. Cerebral edema complicating eclampsia. Am J Obstet Gynecol 2000;182:94.
38. Aukes AM, de Groot JC, Aarnoudse JG, et al. Brain lesions several years after eclampsia. Am J Obstet Gynecol 2009;200(5):504.e1.
39. Postma IR, Wessel I, Aarnoudse JG, et al. Neurocognitive functioning in formerly eclamptic women: sustained attention and executive functioning. Reprod Sci 2009;16:175.
40. Cunningham FG, Fernandez CO, Hernandez C. Blindness associated with preeclampsia and eclampsia. Am J Obstet Gynecol 1995;172:1291.
41. Briggs GG, Freeman RK, Yalfe SJ. Drugs in pregnancy and lactation. 7th edition. Philadelphia: Lippincott Williams and Wilkins; 2005. p. 549.
42. Zondervan HA, Oosting J, Smorenberg-Schoorl ME, et al. Maternal whole blood viscosity in pregnancy hypertension. Gynecol Obstet Invest 1988; 25:83.
43. Jouppila P, Kirkinen P, Koivula A, et al. Labetalol does not alter the placental and fetal blood flow or maternal prostanoids in pre-eclampsia. Br J Obstet Gynaecol 1986;93(6):543.

44. Harper A, Murnaghan GA. Maternal and fetal haemodynamics in hypertensive pregnancies during maternal treatment with intravenous hydralazine or labetalol. Br J Obstet Gynaecol 1991;98(5):453.
45. Sibai BM. Diagnosis and management of gestational hypertension and preeclampsia. Obstet Gynecol 2003;102:181.
46. Ducey JP, Knap KG. Maternal esmolol administration resulting in fetal distress and cesarean section in a term pregnancy. Anesthesiology 1992;77(4):829.
47. Royal College of Obstetricians and Gynaecologists: the management of severe pre-eclampsia. RCOG Guideline 2006;10.
48. Rehman F, Mansour GA, White WB. "Inappropriate" physician habits in prescribing oral nifedipine capsules in hospitalized patients. Am J Hypertens 1996;9:1035.
49. Leveno KJ, Cunningham FG. Management. In: Linheimer MD, Roberts JM, Cunningham FG, editors. Chesley's hypertensive disorders of pregnancy. 3rd edition. New York: Elsevier; 2009. p. 395.
50. Altman D, Carroli G, Duley L, et al. Do women with pre-eclampsia, and their babies, benefit from magnesium sulphate? The Magpie trial: a randomized placebo-controlled trial. Lancet 2002;359(9321):1877.
51. Stempel JE, O'Grady JP, Morton MJ, et al. Use of sodium nitroprusside in complications of gestational hypertension. Obstet Gynecol 1982;60(4):533.
52. Vermillion ST, Scardo JA, Newman RB, et al. A randomized, double-blind trial of oral nifedipine and intravenous labetalol in hypertensive emergencies of pregnancy. Am J Obstet Gynecol 1999;181:858.
53. Magee LA, Cham C, Waterman EJ, et al. Hydralazine for treatment of severe hypertension in pregnancy: meta-analysis. BMJ 2003;327(7421):955.
54. Magee LA, Yong PJ, Espinosa V, et al. Expectant management of severe preeclampsia remote from term: a structured systematic review. Hypertens Pregnancy 2009;28(3):312.
55. Urban G, Vergani P, Ghindini A, et al. State of the art: non-invasive ultrasound assessment of the uteroplacental circulation. Semin Perinatol 2007;31(4):232.
56. Vigil-De Gracia P, Ruiz E, Lopez JC, et al. Management of severe hypertension in the postpartum period with intravenous hydralazine or labetalol: a randomized clinical trial. Hypertens Pregnancy 2007;26(2):163.
57. Scardo JA, Vermillion ST, Newman RB, et al. A randomized, double-blind, hemodynamic evaluation of nifedipine and labetalol in preeclamptic hypertensive emergencies. Am J Obstet Gynecol 1999;181:862.
58. Duley L, Henderson-Smart DJ, Meher S. Drugs for treatment of very high blood pressure during pregnancy. Cochrane Database Syst Rev 2006;(3):CD001449.
59. von Dadelszen P, Magee LA. Fall in mean arterial pressure and fetal growth restriction in pregnancy hypertension: an updated metaregression analysis. J Obstet Gynaecol Can 2002;24(12):941.
60. von Dadelszen P, Ornstein MP, Bull SB, et al. Fall in mean arterial pressure and fetal growth restriction in pregnancy hypertension: a meta-analysis. Lancet 2000;355:87.

Seizures and Intracranial Hemorrhage

Karen L. Wilson, MD*, James M. Alexander, MD

KEYWORDS

- Seizures • Epilepsy • Intracranial hemorrhage • Pregnancy • Aneurysm • Eclampsia
- Stroke • Arteriovenous malformation

KEY POINTS

- Seizures can be detrimental to pregnancy and therefore management of seizures should be aimed at maintaining a seizure-free pregnancy with the lowest dose of medication and avoiding polytherapy when possible.
- Periconceptionual and early obstetric management of women with seizures should include the consideration of preconceptual folate, review of medications and indicated usage, genetic counseling, targeted ultrasound in the presence of anticonvulsant usage, and plans for monitoring anticonvulsant levels during pregnancy.
- Prompt diagnosis of intracerebral hemorrhage by CT or MRI is key because early diagnosis and intervention is pivotal to outcomes.
- Subarachnoid hemorrhage, from either aneurysms or AVMs, is associated with high morbidity and mortality and prompt diagnosis and referral to neurosurgery for management are essential in the first 24 hours from diagnosis.

INTRODUCTION

Seizures are one of the most common neurologic conditions encountered in pregnancy, second only to migraines. It is estimated that seizures complicate up to 0.3% to 0.7% of all pregnancies.[1] In 2005, the Centers for Disease Control and Prevention reported the prevalence of epilepsy in adults as being 1.65%.[2] This estimates more than 1 million women of childbearing age will have a seizure disorder.

Managing seizures in pregnancy can be problematic, because some women have an increase in their seizure activity. Additionally, this disorder can affect fetal development and the course of pregnancy through delivery. Another consideration is the known teratogenic affect of anticonvulsant therapy. Given the physiologic changes in pregnancy, some women may require increased doses of their anticonvulsant or the addition of another anticonvulsant, which may have significant implications to the fetus.[3,4]

Funding Sources: None.
Conflict of Interest: None.
Department of Obstetrics and Gynecology, University of Texas Southwestern Medical Center, 5323 Harry Hines Boulevard, Dallas, TX 75390, USA
* Corresponding author.
E-mail address: KarenL.Wilson@UTSouthwestern.edu

Obstet Gynecol Clin N Am 40 (2013) 103–120
http://dx.doi.org/10.1016/j.ogc.2012.11.009
0889-8545/13/$ – see front matter © 2013 Published by Elsevier Inc.

CAUSES

The most common cause for seizures in pregnancy is prior epilepsy. A small percentage of pregnant women have status epilepticus.[5] Eclampsia is the most common cause for new-onset seizures in pregnancy. In the absence of evidence for preeclampsia or eclampsia, new-onset seizures may be incited by structural and metabolic changes. Structural causes may be from intracranial hemorrhage of various etiologies, cerebral venous sinus thrombosis, ischemic stroke, arteriovenous malformations (AVMs), and brain tumors. Metabolic causes include hyperemesis gravidarum; acute hepatitis from acute fatty liver of pregnancy or viral hepatitis; metabolic diseases; infections; alcohol and drug withdrawal; and electrolyte disturbances, such as hyponatremia, hypoglycemia, or hyperglycemia. Rarely, women can develop gestational epilepsy, in which case the initial seizure occurs in pregnancy and results in recurrent unprovoked seizures. Gestational epilepsy is a diagnosis of exclusion, with the susceptibility most notable in the sixth and seventh months of gestation. After delivery, gestational epilepsy should completely resolve and about half of these women will have seizures in subsequent pregnancies.[6]

PATHOPHYSIOLOGY

Seizures are caused by a paroxysmal event of either abnormal excessive or synchronous neuronal activity in the brain. This abnormal brain activity can be manifested anywhere from dramatic convulsive activity to an experiential phenomenon, not easily discerned by the observer, with or without loss of consciousness. Epilepsy refers to a condition in which a person has recurrent seizures caused by a chronic underlying process and requires the presence of two or more unprovoked seizures. Seizures fall into one of three categories: (1) focal, (2) generalized, or (3) unclassifiable.

Focal seizures arise from a neuronal network that is either discretely localized or broadly distributed within one cerebral hemisphere. Previously, focal seizures had been subcategorized into simple or complex, but they are now classified depending on whether or not there is the presence of cognitive impairment. One can have focal seizure without or with dyscognitive features.

Focal seizures without dyscognitive features can cause motor, sensory, autonomic, or psychic symptoms without cognitive impairment. Features of this type of focal seizure include abnormal motor movement in a very restricted area that can progress to include a larger portion of an extremity or localized paresis for minutes to hours or potentially days. Focal seizures can also result in changes in somatic sensation or autonomic function; alterations in hearing, olfaction, or higher cortical function; and some "internal" feelings.

Focal seizures with dyscognitive features are accompanied by transient impairment of the patient's ability to maintain normal contact with the environment. In this situation, the patient is unable to respond appropriately to visual or verbal commands and has impaired recollection during the ictal phase. These seizures typically begin with an aura.

Generalized seizures involve both cerebral hemispheres and are classified as either typical absence, atypical absence, generalized tonic-clonic, atonic, or myoclonic seizures. Typical absence seizures occur as brief lapses of consciousness without muscle involvement and have a strong genetic component. Generalized tonic-clonic seizures are the most common seizure type in persons with epilepsy, accounting for about 10% of all cases. Generalized seizures are the most commonly associated with metabolic derangements and therefore encountered in many different clinical scenarios.

Lastly, unclassifiable seizures are seizures that cannot be labeled as focal or generalized. They are often manifested as an epileptic spasm, such as a sustained flexion or extension. This occurs predominantly in infants and is likely caused by the immature nature of the central nervous system.

EFFECTS OF EPILEPSY ON PREGNANCY

With improved prenatal care, the seizure-free rate in pregnancy is very high with about two-thirds of women having and improvement or stability of their seizure activity.[7–12] The seizure-free rates can be up to 92% if a woman is seizure-free for at least 9 months to 1 year before pregnancy.[8,11] Further seizure activity in pregnancy does not seem to be affected by the underlying cause, age of the patient, age of seizure onset, and family history of epilepsy.[13,14]

Seizure-free activity during pregnancy can be affected by physiologic changes that occur during the gestational state. This is because anticonvulsant levels can fall as a result of nausea and vomiting in pregnancy; alterations in protein binding and changes in the volume of distribution affecting the unbound versus the total anticonvulsant levels; induction of hepatic, plasma, and placental enzymes that can affect the metabolism of anticonvulsants; increased glomerular filtration that leads to increased renal clearance; decreased intestinal absorption caused by a slower gastrointestinal tract; ingestion of certain drugs (ie, antacids), which may decrease absorption; and compliance by the patient.[5,15,16] Additionally, the seizure threshold can be lowered in pregnancy because of sleep deprivation, hyperventilation of pregnancy, and pain during labor.[17]

In pregnancy, the blood levels of heavily protein-bound drugs fall making it difficult to measure anticonvulsants. Standard anticonvulsant assays determine the total amounts of the drug, free and protein-bound levels, with the latter being the primarily dominant component. Given the fall in plasma protein concentrations in pregnancy, anticonvulsant levels do fall. However, the efficacy of anticonvulsants lie in the unbound level of the drug. This makes standard measurements of anticonvulsants in pregnancy unreliable.[15,18] Total plasma protein levels return to the prepregnancy state within weeks of delivery.[18]

There is controversy regarding current management of anticonvulsant levels. Some current published guidelines recommend monitoring anticonvulsant drug levels every trimester and then 1 month after delivery.[19,20] For those drugs that are highly or moderately bound, such as phenytoin, phenobarbital, carbamazepine, and sodium valproate, it has been recommended to monitor only the drug-free levels.[19,21] Some of the newer anticonvulsants do not have well-established therapeutic ranges, making monitoring difficult. All of this has prompted some organizations to recommend alterations in dosages of anticonvulsants to be based on clinical grounds instead of serum levels.[22]

Another concern is the association between anticonvulsants and malformations in the fetus. It had been suggested that the incidence of malformations in the offspring of women with seizures was two to three times higher than the general population and was a consequence of multifactorial issues and not the effects of anticonvulsants alone.[23–25] Common congenital malformations seen in women with seizures have been orofacial clefts, congenital heart defects, dysmorphic facial features, and neural tube defects. Recent data suggest that the malformation rate in the offspring of women with seizures not on anticonvulsants is similar to the general population, whereas women on anticonvulsants had a significantly higher rate of congenital malformations.[10,26] In women with seizures on anticonvulsants, the rate of congenital malformations was found to be 2.7 to 3.3 times higher and will be discussed in more detail in the next section.[10,26]

Lastly, women with seizures during pregnancy have higher pregnancy complication rates. There has been an association between preeclampsia, growth restriction, post-partum hemorrhage, and respiratory distress in the newborn in women with seizures.[27,28] This complication rate is probably offset in women who are adequately treated for their seizure disorder, as shown in recent studies.[1,10,16] Additionally, women who have uncontrolled seizures are at increased risk for maternal death, up to 5%.[29] Fetal risks associated with uncontrolled maternal seizures may be fetal lactic acidosis, hypoxia, death, and potentially poor cognitive performance in childhood.[7,30–32]

MEDICAL THERAPY DURING PREGNANCY

Most women with seizures need anticonvulsant therapy because there are some defi-nite risks if they have uncontrolled seizures. However, given the teratogenic risks of anticonvulsant therapy, some women discontinue the use of their medication. It is a challenge for the physician to balance the control of a pregnant woman's seizures with the teratogenic risks of the medication. Additionally, physiologic changes in preg-nancy can make it difficult to monitor anticonvulsant drugs in pregnancy.

Several registries have been used to look at the risk of major congenital malforma-tions associated with anticonvulsant therapy.[33–36] Polytherapy with anticonvulsants has demonstrated a significantly higher risk of major congenital malformations, partic-ularly when the combination includes valproic acid.[37] The rate of major congenital mal-formations has been reported up to 15% when valproic acid has been used in conjunction with carbamazepine.[38] However, monotherapy seems to confer a lower risk of teratogenicity, although not negligible. Again, valproic acid is associated with the highest risk of congenital malformation, even when used alone, with rates reported up to 11% or, per the Finnish Medical Birth Registry, a fourfold increase in major congenital malformations.[34]

Other drugs also evaluated in these registries were carbamazepine, lamotrigine, phenobarbital, and phenytoin. Lamotrigine (pregnancy class C drug) is a newer anti-convulsant and has been found to have a relatively low risk of major congenital mal-formations compared with other anticonvulsants with rates reported at 2% to 3%.[33–36] Carbamazepine (pregnancy class D drug) has reported rates of major congenital malformations at 2% to 6%.[33–35] Phenobarbital (pregnancy class D drug), an older anticonvulsant not commonly used as first-line therapy, has demon-strated a risk for major congenital malformations at 6% to 7%.[35,36] Phenytoin (preg-nancy class D drug), another older anticonvulsant, has reported major congenital malformation rates at 3% to 7%.[34–36]

The teratogenicity of the anticonvulsant is likely a dose-dependent effect. When valproic acid was used at 700 to 1500 mg the rates of congenital malformations went from 4.2% to 9% and further rose to 23% when women were taking more than 1500 mg.[36] Similar observations have been made for cabamazepine, lamotrigine, and phenobarbital. It seems prudent to minimize the amount of anticonvulsant taken by a pregnant woman, while being able to maintain her seizure-free status. This further supports checking serum drug levels during pregnancy but only adjusting medication doses based clinical indications. In the event that a seizure occurs, appropriate dose changes can be made.

Other newer anticonvulsants, such as oxcarbazepine, topiramate, gabapentin, and levetiracetam, have only been preliminarily investigated. The sample size is small, but based on initial data these anticonvulsants do not seem to have an increased rate of major congenital malformation when compared with women who had no exposure to anticonvulsant therapy.[11]

In the general population, low folate levels have been associated with neural tube defects and the use of periconceptual supplementation has significantly reduced the incidence of neural tube defects. There have been data to suggest that women with seizures treated with anticonvulsants have low folate levels and this has been linked to an increased risk for adverse pregnancy outcomes.[40,41] The use of folic acid supplementation at 5 to 12 weeks gestation has shown to decrease the incidence of congenital anomalies but it does not eliminate the risk.[42] This area still requires further investigation, but it seems reasonable to recommend periconceptual folic acid supplementation of 0.4 to 5 mg/day to women on anticonvulsants.

GENERAL MANAGEMENT IN PREGNANCY

Women of childbearing age with seizures should be allowed accessible care by an obstetrician.[43] Outside of pregnancy, if a woman has been seizure-free for 2 or more years, then withdrawal of anticonvulsant therapy may be considered. During pregnancy, given that clinicians are unable to predict the likelihood of a seizure occurring, anticonvulsant therapy should be continued. Major convulsions have significant repercussions, such as fetal injury, injury to the mother, and miscarriage.[17] Additionally in pregnancy, monotherapy should be used at the lowest dosages possible. If there is a family history of neural tube defect, then valproic acid and carbamazepine should be avoided, if possible, given the high association with this type of congenital malformation.

During pregnancy, anticonvulsant levels should be monitored on a regular basis. Whenever possible the free, or unbound levels, of the anticonvulsant should be checked. If the levels are low, there is some debate as to whether the dose of the anticonvulsant should be increased if the woman is seizure-free. Without question, if the woman is having seizures then the anticonvulsant therapy should be increased. Given the dose-related risk of major congenital malformations with anticonvulsants, if the anticonvulsant level is low and the woman is seizure-free, it is reasonable to continue to monitor these women without increasing the dosage of their medication. Decreased levels of folate have been described in women on anticonvulsant therapy, particularly phenytoin; therefore, folic acid supplementation is a reasonable recommendation and should be started before conception.[44] Women should be aware that folic acid supplementation does not seem to negate the risk of a congenital malformation. A detailed sonogram should be performed to look at the fetus for any malformations associated with anticonvulsant therapy. In an uncomplicated woman with a history of seizures, tests of fetal well-being are not recommended (**Box 1**).

The development of seizures in pregnancy should be treated immediately, given the risk to the mother and fetus. Women should be placed in the left lateral decubitus

---

Box 1
Preconceptual and Antepartum Management of Women with Seizures

Preconceptual folate supplementation

Maximize seizure-free period prior to conception (9-12 months)

    Avoid valproic acid and carbamazepine, if possible

    Consult to neurology if appropriate

Targeted ultrasound in the presence of anticonvulsant use

Routine monitoring of anticonvulsant serum levels

Avoid analgesics that lower the seizure threshold

position to facilitate fetal blood flow and reduce the risk of aspiration.[45] Then the woman with seizures should receive oxygen, intravenous fluids, and glucose. Electrolytes, complete blood count, calcium, magnesium, glucose, and anticonvulsant drug levels should be obtained. If a woman is on a known anticonvulsant then an additional dose of that medication should be given.[5] If the woman develops status epilepticus, then the drugs of choice are benzodiazepines, diazepam, or clonazepam to try and control the seizures.[15]

During labor, seizures can become more frequent and problematic because of dehydration and sleep deprivation, both of which can lower the seizure threshold. In this scenario, analgesics that also lower the seizure threshold, such as meperidine, should be avoided.[5] If an anticonvulsant is need in labor, then phenytoin can be infused slowly intravenously (<50 mg/min); all anticonvulsants are absorbed rectally and therefore may be given in this fashion (**Box 2**).[15]

THE NEONATE AND BREASTFEEDING

Anticonvulsants can interfere with vitamin K metabolism and neonates can have hemorrhagic disorder of the newborn. Some have recommended vitamin K supplementation in the last month of pregnancy, although this is not likely necessary, and newborns can receive prophylactic vitamin K at delivery. Occasionally, neonates can have some sedation, hyoptonia, poor suckling, and respiratory depression in mothers with high anticonvulsant levels, particularly with barbiturates.[15]

Generally, it is recommended that women with seizures breastfeed and care for their infant like all other mothers. All anticonvulsants are excreted in the breast milk, but at exceedingly low levels, and are dependent on the maternal plasma level. Anticonvulsant levels in the infant depend on their milk intake and absorption, distribution, metabolism, and excretion of the drug.[16] Drug transfer seems to be most extensive with ethosuximide and phenobarbitone, both of which are no longer used with great frequency.[46,47] Data are limited on the newer anticonvulsants, but to date no adverse events have been related to breastfeeding.

PRENATAL COUNSELING

Prenatal counseling should provide some benefit to women with epilepsy, as found in a Cochrane review.[48] This has been questioned by Winterbottom and coworkers,[49]

Box 2
Management of Maternal Seizures

Place mother in left lateral decubitus position

Administer oxygen, intravenous fluids and glucose

Check complete blood count, electrolytes, calcium, magnesium, glucose and anticonvulsant serum level

If on anticonvulsant give an additional dose of that anticonvulsant

If mother develops status epilepticus give either benzodiazipines, diazepam or clonazepam

If mother has eclampsia:

   Treat blood pressure with anti-hypertensives when appropriate

   Give magnesium

If convulsions occur in labor give either phenytoin IV (<50 mg/min) or anticonvulsant rectally who found no objective evidence to its effectiveness. This is a time to address questions that the mother may have and general concerns during pregnancy. Ideally, women should be managed with monotherapy with the least teratogenic drug possible. Furthermore, the obstetrician should stress the importance of compliance with anticonvulsant medication given the significant risks associated to the mother and the fetus with major convulsions. The teratogenic risks should be discussed with the patient and folic acid supplementation may be recommended. Genetic counseling also can be done. In the absence of a family history for epilepsy, the risk for the infant to develop epilepsy is rather low.

INTRACRANIAL HEMORRHAGE

Intracranial hemorrhage is categorized into either intracerebral or subarachnoid hemorrhage (SAH). The underlying cause for each entity is vastly different. In the case of an intracerebral hemorrhage (ICH), typically there is spontaneous rupture of small vessels precipitated by a risk factor. In contrast, SAH is more likely caused by an underlying cerebrovascular malformation in a usually healthy patient. Each entity is discussed next separately.

Intracerebral Hemorrhage

The annual incidence of ICH is 16 to 33 per 100,000[50] and most commonly it is caused by a pathologic underlying condition. It accounts for 10% of all strokes.[51] In pregnancy, the incidence of ICH ranges from 0.01% to 0.05% but is the cause for 5% to 12% of all maternal deaths.[52,53] The most common cause for spontaneous ICH is hypertension and is usually seen in older adults. Besides hypertension, risk factors for ICH include older age, being of African American descent, alcohol or cocaine use, lower cholesterol and lower low-density lipoprotein, and lower triglycerides. Other causes of nontraumatic ICH are amyloid angiopathy, especially in the elderly; vascular malformations; hemorrhagic infarction; septic embolism; mycotic aneurysm; brain tumor; bleeding disorders; infection; moyamoya; and vasculitis. The morbidity and mortality of ICH are extremely high, with mortality reported as high as 80%.[15] In a small case series, 50% of women who developed ICH died, whereas the other half suffered permanent disabilities.[54]

In the setting of hypertension, increased pressure causes spontaneous rupture of small penetrating arteries into the deep part of the brain, near the basal ganglia. Other areas that are frequently affected are the thalamus, cerebellum, and pons. These small arterioles are prone to hypertension-induced vascular injury caused by hypertension-induced degenerative changes in the vessel wall.[55] This was actually first described by Charcot and Bouchard in 1868 who attributed intracerebral bleeding to rupture at the area of microaneurysm.[56] Zeeman and colleagues[57,58] found that cerebral blood flow is significantly increased in preeclampsia. In addition, Zeeman and colleagues[59] found that up to a fourth of women who develop eclampsia suffer from irreversible cerebral ischemia and infarction. This highlights the importance of hypertension management in pregnancy. In the setting of a nonhypertensive patient, other etiologies should be considered, such as hemorrhagic disorders, neoplasms, and vascular malformations.

Presenting symptoms depend on the location of the lesion. ICH generally presents with abrupt neurologic symptoms, whereas seizures are rare. If the lesion is at the putamen, the most common site for hypertensive hemorrhage, then contralateral hemiparesis is the sentinel sign. Thalamic hemorrhages result in contralateral hemiplegia or hemiparesis and can also result in several ocular disturbances. Pontine hemorrhages result in deep coma with quadriplegia. This area can also result in decerebrate rigidity;

pin-point pupils reactive to light; impairment of reflex horizontal eye movements (doll's head); hyperpnea; severe hypertension; and hyperhidrosis. Death is usually imminent except in the case of small hemorrhages. Cerebral and lobar hemorrhages are manifested by headache and vomiting. Cerebellar hemorrhages can also be associated with ataxia. All of these lesions typically progress over time and can result in a diminished level of consciousness and signs of increased intracranial pressures.

Previously, it was generally though that pregnancy increased the risk of ischemic infarction in young women. In the presence of preeclampsia and eclampsia, this is probably true. However, in the general population, studies from Maryland and Washington suggest that the risks of cerebral infarction and ICH are more likely increased during the 6-week period postpartum but not during pregnancy.[60] Another prospective study suggested that women with six or more pregnancies are at an increased risk of ischemic and hemorrhagic stroke.[61]

If ICH is suspected, prompt diagnosis is the key to management. Pregnant women should be managed the same as nonpregnant women given the significant high risk of morbidity and mortality. A comparative study found that magnetic resonance imaging (MRI) was more sensitive than computed tomography (CT) in detecting acute and chronic strokes, but CT still had a similar sensitivity in detecting acute hemorrhagic stroke.[62] Either CT or MRI are reasonable to perform. If a CT scan is negative, but stroke is still suspected, then an MRI can be performed and is better at identifying lesions in the posterior fossa, which may be difficult to see by CT because of bone-induced artifact. MRI can also be used to identify vascular anomalies. The decision on whether CT or MRI is done should take into consideration the cost, proximity to the emergency department, and availability of MRI along with the stability of the patient. Additionally, patients should have blood chemistries and hematologic studies performed, particularly to identify any coagulopathy that may be present.

The mortality with ICH is high; even up to 6 months later the mortality rate is 23% to 58%. Factors predictive of high mortality rate are Glasgow Coma Scale less than 9, volume of hematoma greater than 60 mL, and the presence of ventricular blood.[63–66] The most critical time frame is the first 24 hours after diagnosis, especially the first few hours after diagnosis. About 15% of patients have a continued decline in their Glasgow Coma Scale of greater than or equal to 2 points in the 24 hours after the diagnosis is made.[67]

Early diagnosis and intervention is pivotal. Patients with the diagnosis of ICH should be initially managed in the intensive care unit and appropriate subspecialists should be consulted. A Canadian study demonstrated that patients with ICH managed in the appropriate setting had lower 30-day mortality after adjusting for disease severity, comorbidities, and hospital characteristics.[68]

Further medical management includes correcting any coagulopathy present with the appropriate factor replacement or platelets.[69] If a patient is on warfarin, although not common in pregnant women, these women should receive replacement of vitamin K until the international normalized ratio is corrected.[69] Given the high risk for thromboembolism in patients with ICH, intermittent pneumatic compression with elastic stockings is recommended.[69–72] Less clear is the role of heparin in the prevention of thromboembolism. Studies have not shown a decreased incidence of thromboembolism with the use of heparin but they have also not shown an increase in bleeding when started on Day 4 or Day 10; therefore, the American Heart Association states heparin may be considered in immobile patients 1 to 4 days after diagnosis.[69,73,74]

Blood pressure should be managed accordingly for the pregnant patient. Seizures have been reported in up to 17% of patients with ICH within 2 weeks of the diagnosis.[75–79] Only patients with the presence of clinical seizures should be treated with antiepileptics because a recent analysis demonstrated that antiepileptics, in the absence of clinical seizures, were associated with an increased likelihood of death or disability at 90 days.[80] Patients with a Glasgow Score of less than 9, evidence of transtentorial herniation, or significant intraventricular hemorrhage or hydropcephalus may be considered for intracranial pressure monitoring and treatment.[69]

Surgical risks can be high in these patients and therefore surgical management is only useful in the right clinical setting. Hydrocephalus has been identified as a predictor of ICH morbidity and mortality.[81,82] Therefore, in patients with hydrocephalus and a decreased level of consciousness, ventricular drainage may be used as treatment.[69] Surgical removal of a hematoma may be limited by the location. If the patient has a hematoma larger than 3 cm or brainstem compression or hydrocephalus surgery may be the appropriate management.[83–85] However, if the hematoma is less than 3 cm, there is no brainstem compression, or there is no hydrocephalus, expectant medical management yields reasonable results. If the hematoma is greater than 30 mL and within 1 cm of the cortical surface, then evacuation by craniotomy has shown improved outcomes although not improved survival.[86] However, if the hematoma is greater than 1 cm from the cortical surface or the patient has a Glasgow Score of less than 9, then medical management is the preferable choice.[81] Timing of the surgery must also be taken into consideration. If done too early, there is an increased risk of rebleeding. Therefore, any surgical intervention should probably wait until 12 to 72 hours after diagnosis.[69]

Subarachnoid Hemorrhage

SAH is associated with significant morbidity and mortality. It is the third most common cause of nonobstetric maternal death, with about 90% of those deaths occurring within days of diagnosis, and has an incidence of about 1 to 5 per 10,000 pregnancies.[15] The overall mortality in pregnant women approaches 35%.[87] SAH is more commonly caused by a vascular malformation, such as an intracerebral aneurysm or an AVM, in a relatively healthy patient. Other causes for SAH are hematologic disorders, vasculitides, tumors, venous thromboses, infections, drugs, trauma, and eclampsia. Risk factors for SAH include hypertension, smoking, alcohol and drug abuse, personal or family history of SAH, family history of aneurysms, and certain genetic syndromes.

Intracerebral aneurysm is present in about 5% of the general population, which accounts for up to 10 to 15 million people in the United States, and about 20% to 30% of these patients have multiple aneurysms.[88] Fortunately, most aneurysms do not rupture. Furthermore, aneurysms are not more likely to bleed during pregnancy.[89] If an aneurysm does bleed, they are more likely to bleed during the second half of pregnancy.[87] Presenting symptoms include severe headache with visual changes, cranial nerve abnormalities, focal neurologic deficits, or altered consciousness. Patients can also have signs of meningeal irritation, tachycardia, transient hypertension, low-grade fever, leukocytosis, and proteinuria.

Prompt diagnosis and treatment of SAH from an intracerebral aneurysm is important given the high morbidity and mortality associated with SAH. Noncontrast CT is considered the gold standard for diagnosis, because the sensitivity of CT in the first 3 days after SAH is close to 100%. If it is 5 to 7 days after the diagnosis, it may be necessary to do a lumbar puncture to look for xanthochromia, because the sensitivity of the head CT scan starts to decline at this time. MRI can also be used for diagnosis to avoid lumbar puncture, especially if there is clinical suspicion for SAH and the head CT scan is negative.[90] Clinical severity is the best prognostic indicator and typically assessed by the Hunt and Hess scale.[91,92] Other poor prognostic factors are aneurysm rebleeding, older age, comorbidities, cerebral edema, intraventricular hemorrhage or

ICH, symptomatic vasospasm, delayed cerebral infarction, hyperglycemia, fevers, anemia, and other systemic complications.[90]

Initial management of patients identified with an SAH from an aneurysm should include bed rest, analgesia, sedation, neurologic monitoring, control of blood pressure, and consult to the appropriate specialist. In the nonpregnant patient, the risk of rebleeding is very high within the first 24 hours and has been reported between 4% and 13.6%. Rebleeding is associated with significant morbidity.[93–96] Therefore, prompt treatment should be done if the aneurysm is accessible. In general, pregnant patients with a ruptured aneurysm should be treated the same as nonpregnant patients. Currently, there have been comparisons between microsurgical repair with clipping versus endovascular coil. It seems that endovascular coiling is associated with lower rates of epilepsy and cognitive decline but does have higher rates of rebleeding and incomplete obliteration.[90,97] Decision as to the approach for repair is best left to the neurosurgeon and is based on characteristics of the patient and the aneurysm.

If the aneurysm is occluded and the patient is of good neurologic status, then there is not a neurosurgical contraindication to a pregnant woman having a vaginal delivery. This is not so clear when the aneurysm is occluded within 2 months of delivery. Furthermore, there is some debate as to mode of delivery if a woman has had SAH but has not had surgical repair. Dias and Sekhar[87] did not find a difference in maternal and fetal outcomes in women who underwent cesarean section compared with women who had a vaginal delivery, although the latter group was only comprised of five women. Cartlidge and Shaw[98] recommended against raising the intracranial pressure in women with a ruptured aneurysm that was not surgically repaired, and therefore recommended a cesarean delivery. It seems this may be the more prudent management. A cesarean delivery is also recommended in a woman with an unruptured aneurysm but who is symptomatic.[99] Finally, if an incidental unruptured aneurysm is found and the patient is asymptomatic then cesarean delivery is only indicated for obstetric reasons.[99] To minimize the risk of rupture of the unruptured aneurysm in labor, maternal use of an epidural and a passive second stage of labor (ie, operative delivery with forceps) is recommended.[5,98,99]

AVMs are less common during pregnancy and one study demonstrated only one case in nearly 90,000 deliveries.[100] Pregnancy does not seem to increase the risk of bleeding.[101,102] If bleeding does occur during pregnancy, it can be quite problematic. Most AVMs are congenital, although cases of acquired lesions have been described, and they are shunts that occur between the arterial and venous systems. Most of these hemorrhages are intraparenchymal with about half extending into the subarachnoid space.[51] Typically, bleeding occurs between the ages of 10 and 30 and is more common in males. Symptoms include headache, seizures, and focal neurologic signs. AVMs have an associated morality rate of 6% to 11%.[103]

Most believe that pregnancy does not increase the risk of bleeding from AVM. This was challenged by Dias and Sekhar[87] who reported an increased risk of bleeding with increasing gestational.[102] Pregnant women with an AVM have been reported to have a 3.5% risk of bleeding during pregnancy.[102] In the general population, the risk of hemorrhage increases with individual age and is related to the size of the AVM (volume ≤ 2 cm^3). The peak time of hemorrhage is between the ages 10 and 20 years old, but 40% of all AVMs bleed by age 40 and 72% of those destined to bleed have done so by this time. After an AVM has bled the risk of a second bleed has been reported at about 23% to 34% with an associated mortality rate from the second bleed at around 12% to 13%.[104,105] The overall risk for a rebleed from an AVM is 3.7% per year and there is a risk of death at 0.9% per year.[103]

Initial medical management of SAH in the presence of AVM is the same as for aneurysms. CT or MRI may be used for diagnosis and the first 24 hours is a critical time frame. The efficacy of surgery for these lesions has been unproved to date.[106] In the pregnant patient, neurosurgery considerations are used to assess surgical candidates and the gestational age of the fetus. If the lesion is found in the second trimester, because of the complexity and lengthiness of the surgery, then surgical management may be deferred until after delivery. If surgery is deferred, in the nonpregnant patient, medical therapy includes the use of fibrinolytic and calcium channel blocking agents.[15] Calcium channel blockers have been used in pregnancy without significant adverse effects. In the case of amniocaproic acid, there are few data concerning its use in pregnancy. In the presence of a life-threatening condition and facing the potential loss of the mother, the use of amniocaproic acid may be prudent. In those cases not managed surgically, because of the high risk for rebleeding, cesarean delivery is preferred.[15,107]

ECLAMPSIA

Eclampsia is one of the more common causes for seizures in pregnancy and can result in intracranial hemorrhage (**Box 3**). The rate of eclampsia varies by country, and in general the rates are higher in underdeveloped countries. The latest reviews report an incidence of eclampsia in third-world countries at 91 to 157 per 100,000 deliveries with a case-fatality rate of 6% to 7.5%.[108,109] The incidence of eclampsia in developed countries is significantly lower with rates reported at 1.6 to 10 in 100,000 deliveries with a case-fatality rate of less than 1%.[110–112]

Even though the rate of eclampsia in developed countries has significantly declined over the years, maternal and fetal morbidity and mortality still remain significant. Unfortunately, 38% to 69% of women who develop eclampsia do not typically present with the classic presentation of hypertension and proteinuria, which can make the identification of women at risk for eclampsia difficult.[113,114] The most common prodromal symptom reported in 60% to 80% of these women is headache.[113–115] Other commonly reported prodromal symptoms are visual disturbances and epigastric pain.[113,115] This can make the diagnosis and treatment of women who develop eclampsia challenging.

About half of all eclamptic seizures occur antepartum or intrapartum, whereas the other half occurs postpartum. Most occur within the first 48 hours postpartum and only about 12% occur after this time frame.[114] If the eclamptic seizure occurs outside of the 48 hours postpartum, most occur within 7 days after delivery, but a small number occur up to 42 days postpartum.[114,116] Vigilance and awareness are key in identify and treating these women.

Women with eclampsia have a fourfold increase for cesarean delivery and venous thromboembolism and then have a twofold to threefold increased risk of infection and fetal death. These women are also at significant risk of shock, cardiac arrest, acute respiratory distress syndrome, and renal failure.[110] There can be cerebral damage present and long-term visual dysfunction. Up to 36% of women with eclampsia have the presence of white matter lesions on MRI up to 6 weeks

---

Box 3
Management of Intracranial Hemorrhage

Prompt diagnosis with CT or MRI

Check complete blood count, electrolytes, and coagulation factors

Consider transfer to Intensive Care Unit for monitoring for the first 24 hours after diagnosis

Consult to Neurosurgery

Consider thromboprophylaxis

postpartum. When formerly eclamptic women have these white matter lesions, they have a higher incidence in the decline of their visual quality of life.[117]

The primary key to management is awareness and early diagnosis. Hypertension with a blood pressure of 160/110 should be controlled with the appropriate antihypertensive medication (ie, labetalol or hydralazine).[118] Magnesium should be given immediately. Magnesium is not an anticonvulsant but has an antivasospastic effect. It causes transient lowering of the blood pressure and increased cerebral blood flow and middle cerebral artery perfusion. This lowers the incidence of cerebral ischemia.[119] A very small percentage of women do not respond to magnesium. In that scenario, benzodiazepines or phenytoin have been used.[5] Diagnosis of any coagulopathy or end-organ damage, such as pulmonary edema, should be treated. After the mother is stable, expeditiously delivery of the fetus should be performed.

SUMMARY

Seizures are one of the most common neurologic conditions encountered in pregnancy. The seizure-free rate in pregnancy is highest in women who are seizure-free for 9 to 12 months before pregnancy. The highest rate of congenital malformations is associated with valproic acid or polytherapy and is likely dose-related; therefore, medical therapy should be aimed at the lowest dose of medication and avoiding polytherapy when possible. Breastfeeding is recommended in women with seizures and on anticonvulsants. Periconceptional and early obstetric management of women with seizures should include the consideration of preconceptual folate, review of medications and indicated usage, genetic counseling, targeted ultrasound in the presence of anticonvulsant usage, and plans for monitoring anticonvulsant levels during pregnancy.

Intracranial hemorrhage is caused by intracerebral hemorrhage or SAH. The incidence of intracerebral hemorrhage or SAH is low but is a significant cause of maternal morbidity and mortality. Aneurysms and AVMs are the most common cause of SAH. Aneurysms are not more likely to bleed in pregnancy but if they do bleed it is more likely to occur in the second half of pregnancy. Surgical repair of an aneurysm is not a contraindication to a vaginal delivery. If a pregnant woman has an aneurysm that is not repaired and is symptomatic, she should undergo cesarean delivery. If a pregnant woman has an incidental finding of an aneurysm and is asymptomatic, she can proceed with a vaginal delivery but a passive second stage is recommended. Most AVMs are congenital and women have about a 3.5% risk of bleeding in pregnancy.

Prompt diagnosis of ICH by either CT or MRI is key because early diagnosis and intervention is pivotal to outcomes. Eclampsia is a common cause of seizures in pregnancy and can result in intracranial hemorrhage. The most common prodromal symptom reported for eclampsia is headache.

REFERENCES

1. Richmond JR, Krishnamoorthy P, Andermann E, et al. Epilepsy and pregnancy: an obstetric perspective. Am J Obstet Gynecol 2004;190(2):371–9.
2. Kobau R, Zahran H, Thurman DJ, et al. Epilepsy surveillance among adults—19 states, behavioral risk factor surveillance system. MMWR Surveill Summ 2008; 57(6):1–20.
3. Pennell PB, Peng L, Newport DJ, et al. Lamotrigine in pregnancy. Clearance, therapeutic drug monitoring and seizure frequency. Neurology 2007;70(22 Pt 2): 2130–6.
4. Stefan H, Feurerstein TJ. Novel anticonvulsant drugs. Pharmacol Ther 2007; 113(1):165.

5. Beach RL, Kaplan PW. Seizures in pregnancy: diagnosis and management. Int Rev Neurobiol 2008;83:259–71.
6. Suter C, Lingman WO. Seizure states and pregnancy. Neurology 1956;7:175–9.
7. EURAP Study Group. Seizure control and treatment in pregnancy: observations from EURAP epilepsy pregnancy registry. Neurology 2006;66(3):354–60.
8. Harden CL, Hopp J, Ting TY, et al. Practice parameter update: management issues for women with epilepsy-Focus on pregnancy (an evidence-based review): obstetrical complications and change in seizure frequency. Neurology 2009;73:126–32.
9. Meador KJ, Baker GA, Finnel RH, et al. In utero antiepileptic drug exposure: fetal death and malformations. Neurology 2006;67:407–12.
10. Olafsson E, Hallgrimsson JT, Hauser WA, et al. Pregnancies of women with epilepsy: a population-based study in Iceland. Epilepsia 1998;39(8):887–92.
11. Vajda FJ, Hitchcock A, Graham J, et al. Seizure control in antiepileptic drug-treated pregnancy. Epilepsia 2008;49(1):172–6.
12. Viinikainen K, Heinonen S, Eriksson K, et al. Community-based, prospective controlled study of obstetric and neonatal outcomes of 179 pregnancies in women with epilepsy. Epilepsia 2006;47:186–92.
13. Mattson RH, Cramer JA. Epilepsy, sex hormones and antiepileptic drugs. Epilepsia 1985;26(Suppl 1):S40–51.
14. Levy RH, Yerby MS. Effects of pregnancy on antiepileptic drug utilization. Epilepsia 1985;26(Suppl 1):S52–8.
15. Cartlidge NE. Neurologic disorders. In: Barron WM, Lindheimer MD, Davison JM, editors. Medical disorders during pregnancy. 3rd edition. St Louis (MO): Mosby; 1995. p. 516–39.
16. Battino D, Tomson T. Management of epilepsy during pregnancy. Drugs 2007; 67(18):2727–46.
17. Cunningham FG, Leveno KJ, Bloom SL, et al. Neurological and psychiatric disorders. In: Cunningham FG, Leveno KJ, Bloom SL, et al, editors. Williams obstetrics. 23rd edition. New York: McGraw-Hill; 2010. p. 1164–84.
18. Adab N. Therapeutic monitoring of antiepileptic drugs during pregnancy and in the postpartum period: is it useful? Drugs 2006;20(10):791–800.
19. Practice parameter: management issues for women with epilepsy (summary statement). Report of the Quality Standards Subcommittee of the American Academy of Neurology. Neurology 1998;51(4):944–8.
20. ACOG educational bulletin. Seizure disorders in pregnancy. No 231, 1996. Committee on educational bulletins of the American College of Obstetricians and Gynecologists. Int J Gynaecol Obstet 1997;56:279–86.
21. Vajda F, Solinas C, Graham J, et al. The case for lamotrigine monitoring in pregnancy. J Clin Neurosci 2006;13:103–4.
22. Stokes T, Shaw EJ, Juarez-Garcia A, et al. Clinical guidelines and evidence review for the epilepsies: diagnosis and management in adults and children in primary and secondary care. NICE Clinical Guideline No. CG20. London: Royal College of General Practitioners; 2004.
23. Shapiro S, Hartz SC, Siskind V, et al. Anticonvulsants and parental epilepsy in the development of birth defects (prospective study). Lancet 1976;1(7954): 272–5.
24. Friis ML, Hauge M. Congenital heart defects in live-born children of epileptic parents. Arch Neurol 1985;42(4):374–6.
25. Tomson T, Perucca E, Battino D. Navigating toward fetal and maternal health: the challenge of treating epilepsy in pregnancy. Epilepsia 2004;45(10):1171–5.

26. Fried S, Kozer E, Nulman I, et al. Malformation rates in children of women with untreated epilepsy: a meta-analysis. Drug Saf 2004;27(3):197–202.
27. Pilo C, Wide K, Winbladh B. Pregnancy, delivery, and neonatal complications after treatment with antiepileptic drugs. Acta Obstet Gynecol Scand 2006;85: 643–6.
28. Yerby MS. Epilepsy and pregnancy: new issues for an old disorder. Epilepsy I: diagnosis and treatment. Neurology 1993;11(4):777–86.
29. Cantwell R, Clutton-Brock T, Cooper G, et al. Saving mothers' lives: reviewing maternal deaths to make motherhood safer: 2006-2008. The eight report of the confidential enquiries into maternal deaths in the United Kingdom. BJOG 2011; 188(Suppl 1):1–203.
30. Hiilesmaa VK, Bardy A, Teramo K. Obstetric outcomes in women with epilepsy. Am J Obstet Gynecol 1985;152:499–504.
31. Cummings C, Stewart M, Stevenson M, et al. Neurodevelopment of children exposed in utero to lamotrigine, sodium valproate and carbamazepine. Arch Dis Child 2011;96:643–7.
32. Meador KJ, Baker GA, Browning N, et al. Cognitive function at 3 years of age after fetal exposure to antiepileptic drugs. N Engl J Med 2009;360(16): 1597–605.
33. Artama M, Auviene A, Raudaskoski T, et al. Antiepileptic drug use of women with epilepsy and congenital malformations in offspring. Neurology 2005;64:1874–8.
34. Cunnington MC, Weil JG, Messenheimer JA, et al. Final results from 18 years of the international lamotrigine pregnancy registry. Neurology 2011;76:1817–23.
35. Morrow J, Russel A, Guthrie E, et al. Malformation risks of antiepileptic drugs in pregnancy: a prospective study from the UK epilepsy and pregnancy register. J Neurol Neurosurg Psychiatry 2006;77:193–8.
36. Tomson T, Battino D, Bonizzoni E, et al. Dose-dependent risk of malformations with antiepileptic drugs: an analysis of data from the EURAP epilepsy and pregnancy registry. Lancet Neurol 2011;10:609–17.
37. Meador K, Reynolds MW, Cream S, et al. Pregnancy outcomes in women with epilepsy: a systematic review and meta-analysis of published pregnancy registries and cohorts. Epilepsy Res 2008;81:1–13.
38. Holmes LB, Mittendorf R, Shen A, et al. Fetal effects of anticonvulsant polytherapies: different risks from different drug combinations. Arch Neurol 2011;64:961–5.
39. Molgaard-Nielsen D, Hviid A. Newer-generation antiepileptic drugs and risk of major birth defects. JAMA 2011;305:1996–2002.
40. Hiilesmaa VK, Teramo K, Granstrom ML, et al. Serum folate concentrations during pregnancy in women with epilepsy: relation to antiepileptic drug concentrations, number of seizures, and fetal outcome. Br Med J (Clin Res Ed) 1983; 287(6392):577–9.
41. Dansky LV, Andermann E, Rosenblatt D, et al. Anticonvulsants, folate levels, and pregnancy outcome: a prospective study. Ann Neurol 1987;21(2):176–82.
42. Kjaer D, Horvath-Puho E, Christensen J, et al. Antiepileptic drug use, folic acid supplementation, and congenital abnormalities: a population-based case-control study. BJOG 2008;115:98–103.
43. Crawford P, Appleton R, Betts T, et al. Best practice guidelines for the management of women with epilepsy. Seizure 1999;8:201–17.
44. Neural tube defects. ACOG practice bulletin No. 44. American College of Obstetricians and Gynecologists. Obstet Gynecol 2003;102:203–13.
45. Barnett C, Richens A. Epilepsy and pregnancy: report of an Epilepsy Research Foundation Workshop. Epilepsy Res 2003;52:147–87.

46. Kuhnz W, Koch S, Jakob S, et al. Ethosuximide in epileptic women during pregnancy and lactation period: placental transfer, serum concentrations in nursed infants and clinical status. Br J Clin Pharmacol 1984;18(5):671–7.
47. Kuhnz W, Koch S, Helge H, et al. Primidone and phenobarbital during lactation period in epileptic women: total and free drug serum levels in the nursed infants and their effects on neonatal behavior. Dev Pharmacol Ther 1988;11(3):147–54.
48. Adab N, Tudur SC, Vineten J, et al. Common antiepileptic drugs in pregnancy in women with epilepsy. Cochrane Database Syst Rev 2004;(3):CD004848.
49. Winterbottom J, Smyth R, Jacoby A, et al. The effectiveness of preconception to reduce adverse pregnancy outcome in women with epilepsy: what's the evidence? Epilepsy Behav 2009;14(2):273–9.
50. Sacco S, Marini C, Toni D, et al. Incidence and 10-year survival of intracerebral hemorrhage in a population-based registry. Stroke 2009;40:394–9.
51. Smith WS, English JD, Johnston SC. Cerebrovascular diseases. In: Longo DL, Fauci AS, Kasper DL, et al, editors. Harrison's principles of internal medicine. 18th edition. New York: McGraw-Hill; 2012.
52. Pumar JM, Pardo MI, Carreira JM, et al. Endovascular treatment of an acutely ruptured intracranial aneurysm in pregnancy: report of eight cases. Emerg Radiol 2010;17:205–7.
53. Berg CJ, Gallaghan WM, Syverson C, et al. Pregnancy-related mortality in the United States, 1998 to 2005. Obstet Gynecol 2010;116(6):1302–9.
54. Martin JN Jr, Thigpen BD, Moore RC, et al. Stroke and severe preeclampsia and eclampsia: a paradigm shift focusing on systolic blood pressure. Obstet Gynecol 2005;105(2):246–54.
55. Takebayashi S, Kaneko M. Electron microscopic studies of ruptured arteries in hypertensive intracerebral hemorrhage. Stroke 1983;14:28–36.
56. Qureshi AI, Tuhrim S, Broderick JP, et al. Spontaneous intracerebral hemorrhage. N Engl J Med 2001;344(19):1450–60.
57. Zeeman GG, Hatab MR, Twickler DM. Maternal cerebral blood flow changes in pregnancy. Am J Obstet Gynecol 2003;189(4):968–72.
58. Zeeman GG, Hatab MR, Twickler DM. Increased cerebral blood flow in preeclampsia with magnetic resonance imaging. Am J Obstet Gynecol 2004;191:1425–9.
59. Zeeman GG, Fleckenstein JL, Twickler DM, et al. Cerebral infarction in eclampsia. Am J Obstet Gynecol 2004;190:714–20.
60. Kittner SJ, Stern BJ, Feeser BR, et al. Pregnancy and the risk of stroke. N Engl J Med 1996;335:768–74.
61. Qureshi AI, Giles WH, Croft JB, et al. Number of pregnancies and risk for stroke and stroke subtypes. Arch Neurol 1997;54:203–6.
62. Chalela JA, Kidwell CS, Nentwich LM, et al. Magnetic resonance imaging and computed tomography in emergency assessment of patients with suspected acute stroke: a prospective comparison. Lancet 2007;369:293–8.
63. Qureshi AI, Safdar K, Weil J, et al. Predictors of early deterioration and mortality in black Americans with spontaneous intracerebral hemorrhage. Stroke 1995;26:1764–7.
64. Broderick JP, Brott TG, Buldner JE, et al. Volume of intracerebral hemorrhage: a powerful and easy-to-use predictor of 30-day mortality. Stroke 1993;25:987–93.
65. Lisk DR, Pasteur W, Rhoades H, et al. Early presentation of hemispheric intracerebral hemorrhage: prediction of outcome and guidelines for treatment allocation. Neurology 1994;44:133–9.

66. Tuhrim S, Horowitz DR, Sacher M, et al. Validation and comparison of models predicting survival following intracerebral hemorrhage. Crit Care Med 1994; 23:950–4.
67. Brott T, Broderick J, Kothari R, et al. Early hemorrhage growth in patients with intracerebral hemorrhage. Stroke 1997;28:1–5.
68. Diringer MN, Edwards DR. Admission to a neurologic/neurosurgical intensive care unit is associated with reduced mortality rate after intracerebral hemorrhage. Crit Care Med 2001;29:635–40.
69. Morgensten LB, Hemphill JC III, Anderson C, et al. Guidelines for the management of spontaneous intracerebral hemorrhage: a guideline for healthcare professional from the American Heart Association/American Stroke Association. Stroke 2010;41:2108–29.
70. Gregory PC, Kuhlemeier KV. Prevalence of venous thromboembolism in acute hemorrhagic and thromboembolic stroke. Am J Phys Med Rehabil 2003;83:364–9.
71. Kawase K, Okazaki S, Toyoda K, et al. Sex difference in the prevalence of deep-vein thrombosis in Japanese patients with acute intracerebral hemorrhage. Cerebrovasc Dis 2009;27:313–9.
72. Christensen MC, Dawson J, Vincent C. Risk of thromboembolic complications after intracerebral hemorrhage according to ethnicity. Adv Ther 2008;25:831–41.
73. Boeer A, Voth E, Henze T, et al. Early heparin therapy in patients with spontaneous intracerebral haemorrhage. J Neurol Neurosurg Psychiatry 1991;54:466–7.
74. Dickmann U, Voth E, Schicha H, et al. Heparin therapy, deep-vein thrombosis and pulmonary embolism after intracerebral hemorrhage. Klin Wochenschr 1988;66:1182–3.
75. Berger AR, Lipton RB, Lesser ML, et al. Early seizures following intracerebral hemorrhage: implications for therapy. Neurology 1988;38:1363–5.
76. Bladin CF, Alexandrov AV, Bellavance A, et al. Seizures after stroke: a prospective multicenter study. Arch Neurol 2000;57:1617–22.
77. Passero S, Rocchi R, Rossi S, et al. Seizures after spontaneous supratentroial intracerebral hemorrhage. Epilepsia 2002;43:1175–80.
78. Sung CY, Chu NS. Epileptic seizures in intracerebral haemorrhage. J Neurol Neurosurg Psychiatry 1989;52:1273–6.
79. Yang TM, Lin WC, Chang WN, et al. Predictors and outcome of seizures after spontaneous intracerebral hemorrhage. J Neurosurg 2009;111:87–93.
80. Messe SR, Sansing LH, Cucchiara BL, et al. CHANT investigators. Prophylactic antiepileptic drug use is associated with poor outcome following ICH. Neurocrit Care 2009;11:38–44.
81. Bhattathiri PS, Gregson B, Prasad KS, et al. STICH Investigators. Invtraventricular hemorrhage and hydrocephalus after spontaneous intracerebral hemorrhage: results from the STICH trial. Acta Neurochir Suppl 2006;96:65–8.
82. Diringer MN, Edwards DR, Zazulia AR. Hydrocephalus: a previously unrecognized predictor of poor outcome from supratentorial intracerebral hemorrhage. Stroke 1998;29:1352–7.
83. Da Pian R, Bazzan A, Pasqualin A. Surgical versus medical treatment of spontaneous posterior fossa haematomas: a cooperative study in 205 cases. Neurol Res 1984;6:145–51.
84. Kirollos RW, Tyagi AK, Ross SA, et al. Management of spontaneous cerebellar hematomas: a prospective treatment protocol. Neurosurgery 2001;49:1378–86.
85. Morioka J, Fujii M, Kato S, et al. Japan Standard Stroke Registry Group (JSSR). Surgery for spontaneous intracerebral hemorrhage has greater remedial value than conservative therapy. Surg Neurol 2006;65:67–72.

86. Pantazis G, Tsitsopoulos P, Mihas C, et al. Early surgical treatment vs conservative management for spontaneous supratentorial intracerebral hematomas: a prospective randomized study. Surg Neurol 2006;66:492–501.

87. Dias MS, Sekhar LN. Intracranial hemorrhage from aneurysms and ateriovenous malformations during pregnancy and the pueperium. Neurosurgery 1990;27(6): 855–65.

88. Singer RJ, Ogilvy CS, Rordorf G. Etiology, clinical manifestations, and diagnosis of aneurismal subarachnoid hemorrhage. UpToDate; 2012.

89. Roman H, Descargues G, Lopes M. Subarachnoid hemorrhage due to cerebral aneurismal rupture during pregnancy. Acta Obstet Gynecol Scand 2004;83: 330–4.

90. Connolly ES Jr, Rabinstein AA, Carhuapoma JR, et al. Guidelines for the management of aneurysmal subarachnoid hemorrhage: a guideline for healthcare professional from the American Heart Association/American Stroke Association. Stroke 2012;43:1711–37.

91. Hunt WE, Hess RM. Surgical risk as related to time of intervention in the repair of intracranial aneurysms. J Neurosurg 1968;28:14–20.

92. Report of World Federation of Neurological Surgeons Committee on a universal subarachnoid hemorrhage grading scale. J Neurosurg 1988;68:985–6.

93. Hillman J, Fridriksson S, Nilsson O, et al. Immediate administration of tranexamic acid and reduced incidence of early rebleeding after aneurismal subarachnoid hemorrhage: a prospective randomized study. J Neurosurg 2002;97:771–8.

94. Kassell NF, Torner JC. Aneurysmal rebleeding: a preliminary report from the Cooperative Aneurysm Study. Neurosurgery 1983;13:479–81.

95. Naidech AM, Janjua N, Kreiter KT, et al. Predictors and impact of aneurysm rebleeding after subarachnoid hemorrhage. Arch Neurol 2005;62:410–6.

96. Ohkuma H, Tsurutani H, Suzuki S. Incidence and significance of early aneurismal rebleeding before neurosurgical or neurological management. Stroke 2002;32: 1176–80.

97. Molyneux AJ, Kerr RS, Yu LM, et al. International Subarachnoid Aneurysm Trial (ISAT) collaborative Group, International Subarachnoid Aneurysm Trial (ISAT) of neurosurgical clipping versus endovascular coiling in 2143 patients with ruptured intracranial aneurysms: a randomized comparison of effects on survival, dependency, seizures, rebleeding, subgroups, and aneurysm occlusion. Lancet 2005; 366:809–17.

98. Cartlidge NE, Shaw DA. Intrasellar aneurysm with subarachnoid hemorrhage and hypopituitarism. Case report. J Neurosurg 1972;36(5):640–3.

99. Stoodley MA, Macdonald RL, Weir BK. Pregnancy and intracranial aneurysms. Neurosurg Clin N Am 1998;9(3):549–56.

100. Simolke GA, Cox SM, Cunningham FG. Cerebrovascular accident complicating pregnancy and the puerperium. Obstet Gynecol 1991;78:37–42.

101. Finnerty JJ, Chisholm CA, Chapple H, et al. Cerebral arteriovenous malformation in pregnancy: presentation and neurologic, obstetric, and ethical significance. Am J Obstet Gynecol 1999;181:296–303.

102. Horton JC, Chambers WA, Lyons SL, et al. Pregnancy and the risk of hemorrhage from cerebral arteriovenous malformations. Neurosurgery 1990;27:867–72.

103. Wilkins RH. Natural history of intracranial vascular malformations: a review. Neurosurgery 1985;16(3):421–30.

104. Perret G, Nishioka H. Ateriovenous malformations: an analysis of 545 cases of cranio-cerebral arteriovenous malformations and fistulae reported to the Cooperative Study. J Neurosurg 1966;25:467–90.

105. Svien HJ, McRae JA. Arteriovenous anomalies of the brain: fate of the patients not having definitive surgery. J Neurosurg 1965;23(1):23–8.
106. Fewel ME, Thompson BG, Hoff JT. Spontaneous intracerebral hemorrhage: a review. Neurosurg Focus 2003;15(4):1–16.
107. Friedlander RM. Ateriovenous malformations of the brain. N Engl J Med 2007; 356(26):2704–12.
108. Miguil M, Chekairi A. Eclampsia: study of 342 cases. Hypertens Pregnancy 2008;27:203–11.
109. Eke AC, Ezebiabe IU, Okafor C. Presentation and outcome of eclampsia at a tertiary center in South East Nigeria: a 6-year review. Hypertens Pregnancy 2011;30:125–32.
110. Liu S, Joseph KS, Liston KM, et al. Incidence, risk factors, and associated complications of eclampsia. Obstet Gynecol 2011;118(5):987–94.
111. Tan KH, Kwek K, Yeo GS. Epidemiology of preeclampsia and eclampsia at KK Women's and Children's Hospital, Singapore. Singapore Med J 2006;47:48–53.
112. Sibai BM. Diagnosis, prevention, and management of eclampsia. Obstet Gynecol 2005;105:402–10.
113. Douglas K, Redman CW. Eclampsia in the United Kingdom. BMJ 1996;309: 1395–400.
114. Al-Safi Z, Imudia AN, Filetti LC, et al. Delayed postpartum preeclampsia and eclampsia: demographics, clinical course and complications. Obstet Gynecol 2011;118(5):1102–7.
115. Cooray SC, Edmond SM, Tong S, et al. Characterization of symptoms immediately preceeding eclampsia. Obstet Gynecol 2011;118:987–94.
116. Roberts JM, Redman CW. Preeclampsia: more than pregnancy-induced hypertension. Lancet 1993;341:1447–51.
117. Weigman MJ, Groot JC, Jansonius NM, et al. Long-term visual functioning after eclampsia. Obstet Gynecol 2012;119(5):959–66.
118. Cunningham FG. Severe preeclampsia and eclampsia: systolic hypertension is also important. Obstet Gynecol 2005;105(2):237–8.
119. Belfort MA, Moise KJ. Effect of magnesium sulfate on maternal brain flow in preeclampsia: a randomized placebo controlled study. Am J Obstet Gynecol 1992;167:661–6.

Endocrine Emergencies

Scott A. Sullivan, MD, MSCR*, Christopher Goodier, MD

KEYWORDS

- Thyroid storm • Diabetic ketoacidosis (DKA) • Hypoparathyroidism
- Myxedematous coma • Pregnancy endocrinopathies

KEY POINTS

- Thyroid Storm in pregnancy is a true obstetric emergency with significant fetal and maternal morbidity and even mortality. Prompt recognition and aggressive treatment are the keys to maximizing outcome for both patients.
- Diabetic ketoacidosis is also a serious obstetric emergency with significant fetal morbidity and mortality. Fetal demise and preterm birth are not unusual in this scenario. Fluid replacement, insulin therapy, and electrolyte replacement and management are keys to maternal supportive care and successful fetal resuscitation.
- Hyperparathyroidism is a relatively rare but potentially serious cause of hypercalcemia. Severe hypercalcemia can result in generalized tetany and maternal cardiovascular complications. Supportive care is an important element for management but ultimately localization and removal of the source of excess parathyroid hormone is curative.

THYROID STORM

Thyroid storm is a potentially fatal endocrine emergency characterized by a severe hypermetabolic state precipitated by high levels of endogenous thyroid hormones. The use of the word "storm" describes both the intensity of the clinical presentation and the significance of the elevations of both thyroxine (T4) and tri-iodothyronine (T3). Most cases are a result of poorly controlled hyperthyroidism, although there are cases of unrecognized and rapidly progressive hyperthyroidism. Rates of case fatality vary in different series, but range from 10% to 30%.[1] Rapid recognition, prompt supportive care, and intervention likely maximize maternal and fetal outcomes.

The exact triggering mechanism for thyroid storm is unknown. A significant number of cases have no identifiable antecedent cause other than preexisting hyperthyroidism. Graves disease, or the presence of thyroid-stimulating antibodies, is the most common underlying cause of hyperthyroidism in pregnancy. Thyroid storm may also be associated with certain preceding events, such as infection, surgery, trauma, venous thromboembolism, and other endocrinopathies, such as diabetic ketoacidosis.[2]

Dept of Obstetrics and Gynecology, 96 Jonathan Lucas Street, Charleston, SC 29466, USA
* Corresponding author.
E-mail address: sullivas@musc.edu

Obstet Gynecol Clin N Am 40 (2013) 121–135
http://dx.doi.org/10.1016/j.ogc.2012.12.001
0889-8545/13/$ – see front matter © 2013 Published by Elsevier Inc.

obgyn.theclinics.com

Thyroid receptors are present in most tissues, and thyroid hormones exert many different regulatory influences throughout the body.[3] T3 is the most active hormone and may be produced primarily in the thyroid gland or through peripheral deiodination. The thyroid gland sits in the anterior neck and is comprised of lobules, which house the follicles where iodine is trapped and thyroid hormones are processed (**Fig. 1**). Peripheral conversion occurs in many tissues but is most prevalent in the skeletal muscle, liver, and cardiac tissues. T3 targets the nuclear receptors as well as mitochondria inside the cell. Excess T3 stimulation can lead to increased lipolysis, cardiac output, increased oxygen consumption, and heat production.

Presenting signs and symptoms can be variable and are summarized in **Box 1**. They commonly include tachycardia, diaphoresis, anxiety or confusion, weakness, hyperpyrexia, and a widened pulse pressure.[4] The presentation may be nonspecific enough to be confused with any number of other conditions, which may lead to a delay in diagnosis and treatment. Infection and sepsis often will be considered as a competing diagnosis given the high temperature and pulse. They may be coexistent with thyroid storm as well. A prominent goiter, thyroid bruit, or exopthalmos may be discriminating physical signs that are more specific to thyroid dysfunction.

Laboratory analysis may be useful in making a diagnosis, especially in patients who have no reported history of thyroid dysfunction or in those who cannot communicate. Thyroid-stimulating hormone is usually undetectable, although cautious interpretation is required in the first trimester because of the suppressive effects of human chorionic

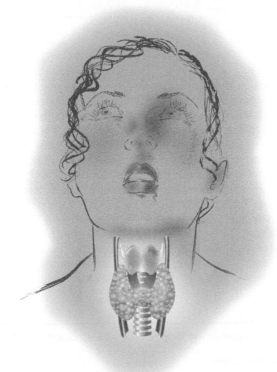

Fig. 1. The usual anatomic location of the normal human thyroid gland.

Box 1
Signs and symptoms of thyroid storm

Tachycardia	Goiter
Hyperpyrexia	Exopthalmos
Tachypnea	Diaphoresis
Hypoxia	Chest pain
Tremors	Palpitations
Confusion	Atrial fibrillation
Agitation	Nausea/vomiting
Pulmonary edema	Anorexia
Fetal tachycardia	Visual changes

---

gonadotropin. Free T4 and free T3 are often well above the upper limits of normal in pregnancy. Levels of total hormone are also usually elevated. Trimester and laboratory-specific reference ranges should be used. However, there are no generally accepted levels at which the diagnosis of thyroid storm is assured, and there may be significant laboratory overlap with simple hyperthyroidism. The white blood cell count may be variably elevated. There may also be evidence of dehydration, acidosis, hyperglycemia, hypercalcemia, elevated liver enzymes, and electrolyte disturbances on metabolic panel screening.

Burch and Wartofsky have outlined a commonly cited clinical scoring system for the probability of thyroid storm.[5] Points are allocated for elevation in temperature, maternal pulse, and several organ system dysfunctions. Scores can indicate a high, medium, or low probability of the diagnosis of thyroid storm. Imaging is of limited benefit, as thyroid scans can be time consuming and nonspecific. Chest radiographs and computed tomographic scans can be useful when looking for concomitant infections or pulmonary pathologic abnormalities, such as edema or emboli. Primarily, it remains a clinical and somewhat arbitrary diagnosis.[4]

The maternal adaptations to pregnancy are also factors that must be considered when making the diagnosis of thyroid storm. Mild tachycardia and leukocytosis are not unusual in pregnancy. Pre-eclampsia may present with hypertension, systemic symptoms, pulmonary edema, and even heart failure. Interpretation of maternal acid-base status must take into consideration the moderate compensated respiratory alkalosis that occurs in pregnancy. The fetus is also likely to respond to the maternal derangements of metabolism. Fetal tachycardia, or >180 beats per minute, is frequently present. Along with tachycardia, there can be loss of variability in baseline changes. Maternal acidosis may also lead to fetal acidosis and resulting changes in fetal heart tracings, including late decelerations. Fetal morbidity remains high with thyroid storm, with significant incidences of preterm birth, neonatal complications, and even fetal death.[6]

A diagnosis of thyroid storm requires prompt intervention for both mother and fetus. Care should be multidisciplinary, potentially involving Maternal-Fetal Medicine, Endocrinology, or Critical Care specialists. Most patients would benefit from management in an intensive care setting, with the availability of continuous fetal monitoring if the fetus has reached a survivable gestational age. In general, every effort should be made to resuscitate the mother before considering delivery for fetal indications.[7] However, the presence of a persistent fetal bradycardia or the development of category III heart rate tracing that is unresponsive to resuscitative measures may require expedited delivery for a viable fetus.

Immediate treatment steps require the placement of adequate intravenous access, replacement of fluids, interpretation of heart rhythm, and ensuring oxygenation **(Fig. 2)**. Arrhythmias, such as atrial fibrillation, may be present in a minority of patients but require monitoring and treatment. Electrocardiogram or telemetry is recommended. Respiratory failure is a late finding, but intubation and mechanical ventilation are sometimes necessary. Poor pulmonary function may be reflected in fetal response as well. Simultaneous assessment of several organ systems, including the fetus, is required.

Definitive treatment of thyroid storm also involves the use of several medications in addition to supportive care. The mainstays of antithyroid medications are the thionamides. In the United States, this consists of propothiourocil (PTU) and methimazole.[8] Both agents act within the thyroid gland to inhibit follicular growth and development and the packaging of iodothyronines into T4 and T3. One advantage of PTU is that in addition to the antithyroid effects within the gland it also inhibits peripheral conversion at the tissue level of T4 to T3, which limits the active form of thyroid hormone. However, there is a significant disadvantage to the use of PTU in that there have been rare cases of fulminate liver failure and death associated with its use, including instances in pregnancy. There is a Food and Drug Administration "black box" warning

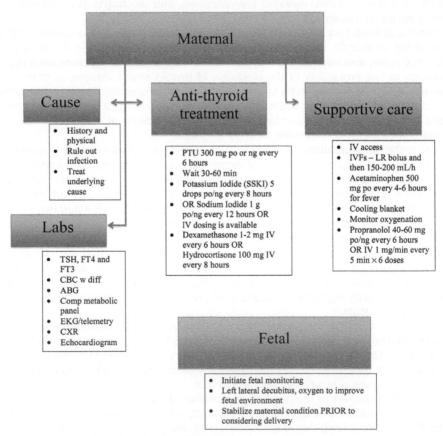

Fig. 2. Treatment algorithm for thyroid storm.

for PTU concerning this link to hepatotoxicity. It is unclear how thyroid storm specifically affects this risk.

Methimazole use in pregnancy has been linked to some teratogenic effects including aplasia cutis.[9] This association is not particularly strong in the literature so its use is generally considered to be acceptable, especially outside the time of organogenesis. In addition, a life-threatening agranulocytosis may rarely develop after methimazole use. Given these conflicting risks, there is no clear recommendation for which thionamide to initiate in a thyroid storm. **Box 2** summarizes the recommended doses of commonly used medications in a thyroid storm.

In addition to thionamide use to decrease the production of T3 and T4, it is also recommended to use iodide-containing medication to inhibit the further release of active thyroid hormone from the thyroid gland. Oral potassium iodide, 5 drops every 8 hours, or sodium iodide 1000 mg intravenously (IV) every 12 hours may be used. It is generally thought that the iodines should not be administered before the use of thionamides for the risk of an unintended release of thyroid hormones from the thyroid. The general time frame is recommended to be 30 to 60 minutes after the initiation of thionamides.[8]

Corticosteroids can also be administered that have the effect of decreasing systemic inflammation as well as peripheral effects of decreasing T4 to T3 conversion. Other supportive medications include antipyretics, such as acetaminophen and β-blockade.

Considering that high-output cardiac failure is one of the leading causes of mortality in a thyroid storm, the judicious use of a β- blockade may be one of the most important of the thyroid storm medications. Labetalol, atenolol, or propranolol may be used for rate and output control. Propanolol also reduces T4 to T3 conversion. Long-term use of β-blockers has been associated with fetal growth restriction but is generally considered safe in a risk/benefit consideration.

Conventional treatments may fail after trials of medical management in the most severe cases. There also may be adverse reactions to the thionamides, which may require discontinuation. Emergency thyroidectomy, with or without plasmaphoresis, has been described successfully in thyroid storm, but must be considered a high-risk undertaking.[10]

MYXEDEMATOUS COMA (SEVERE HYPOTHYROIDISM)

Myxedematous coma is a rare condition characterized by severe hypothyroidism with multiple systemic effects. It is roughly the equivalent of thyroid storm for

---

Box 2
Treatment options for hyperparathyroidism/hypercalcemia

Hydration

    Isotonic saline @ 200 mL/h

Increasing excretion

    Calcitonin 4 IU/kg sq every 6 hours

Diuresis

    Lasix 20–40 mg IV*

Inhibiting PTH

    Cinacalcet 30 mg po bid

* Used only for fluid overload

hypothyroidism. The exact incidence is unknown with only a few hundred cases reported in the literature. There are cases that have been reported in pregnancy.[11]

The term myxedematous coma refers to 2 of the more common clinical signs associated with the condition. A generalized edema, especially of the lower extremities, has been coined myxedema. The addition of the term coma is somewhat misleading in that the patient does not have to be comatose to carry this diagnosis. Mental status changes are very common but may be limited to confusion, agitation, memory loss, or combativeness. Other symptoms associated with myxedematous coma are somnolence, cardiac arrhythmias, multiorgan system failure, headaches, nausea and vomiting, temperature instability, and hypotension.

The diagnosis may be difficult based on the rarity of the condition as well as the lack of specificity among many of the early symptoms. Pregnancy can frequently be complicated by fatigue, weight changes, changes in temperature perception, and aberrations in sleeping. However, clinical suspicion must be maintained, especially among patients with compelling histories of hypothyroidism. Hashimoto thyroiditis is the most common associated cause of hypothyroidism along with autoimmune hypothyroidism. Postablation hypothyroidism should not be ignored because the level of hypothyroidism may change over time and patients may be under the mistaken impression that they are cured and no longer need to monitor their thyroid status.

Typically, thyroid function tests will be significantly aberrant in this condition. A very high thyroid-stimulating hormone and a very low free T4 and free T3 are anticipated. However, there can be a significant amount of variation in what is observed. Treatment is similar to a thyroid storm, consisting of both supportive care as well as specific treatment targeting the disease. Supportive care would include admission to the hospital and possibly to the intensive care unit, close attention to cardiac arrhythmias, electrolyte balance, fluid balance, and fetal status. The mental status changes should be monitored and any precautions, such as fall precautions, not leaving the patient alone, and enlisting the help of family members in the care of the patient, are prudent.

Corticosteroid use may decrease the systemic symptoms while awaiting the effect of thyroid replacement. Because the cause of the condition is severe lack of thyroid hormones, the ultimate treatment is thyroid replacement.[12] However, it may take a significant amount of time and several days to replace adequately what has been lost. The supportive care must continue until adequate levels have been repleted. Typical doses of levothyroxine are 200 to 250 mg per day IV. Oral replacement has also been described in other circumstances. Most obstetricians and gynecologists do not have experience with replacing thyroid hormones via the intravenous route. A consultation with Endocrinology and/or Critical Care specialists is recommended.

DIABETIC KETOACIDOSIS

Diabetic ketoacidosis (DKA) is a medical emergency that remains one of the most serious complications that occurs in pregnancy. It can result in both maternal and fetal morbidity and mortality. Importantly, the overall incidence of DKA in pregnancy has decreased from approximately 10% to 20% in the late 1970s to approximately 1% to 2% in most recent reports.[3,13,14] The improvement has been attributed to early recognition and aggressive multidisciplinary management and has resulted in a decreased maternal rate of mortality from approximately 5% to 15% to now approximately 1%. Rate of fetal mortality has also improved from a reported rate of 50% to 85% to approximately 9%.[3,13–15] Preterm birth, from both premature labor and medical intervention, is a common sequelae from severe DKA.

The pathophysiology of DKA is the result of a complex interplay in which inadequate insulin action results in perceived hypoglycemia at the cellular level of target cells, such as those in the liver, adipose, and muscle tissues (**Fig. 3**). The body responds with an exaggerated counterregulatory response, principally releasing glucagon, which worsens the already significant level of hyperglycemia in the serum, causing osmotic diuresis and resultant dehydration, profound hypovolemia, and electrolyte depletion.

The lack of insulin and production of counterregulatory hormones in the adipose tissue activates hormone-sensitive lipase, which causes the release of free fatty acids into the circulation, which are ultimately oxidized to ketone bodies, including acetoacetate, 3-β-hydroxybutyrate, and acetone. It is the acetone formation that yields the characteristic fruity breath odor in DKA. Acidosis occurs secondary to ketone body formation, which contributes to a large pool of hydrogen ions. These ions can overwhelm the buffering capacity of the body, leading to a metabolic acidosis manifested as an anion gap. Keto acids bind sodium and potassium, which are excreted in the urine, further worsening the electrolyte balance. The final common pathway if this process is left untreated can lead to cardiac dysfunction, decreased tissue perfusion, and worsened renal function, leading to shock, coma, and death.[3,16]

The normal physiologic changes of pregnancy increase the susceptibility of the gravid parturient to DKA. Pregnancy constitutes a diabetogenic state secondary to impaired action of maternal insulin primarily because of the action of human placental

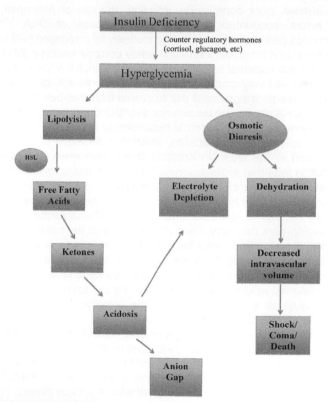

Fig. 3. Pathophysiology of DKA.

lactogen and progesterone, as well as increased production of placental insulinase. Thus, the normal exogenous insulin requirements increase with advancing gestation during pregnancy for diabetic mothers, predisposing them to DKA.

In addition, respiratory adaptations of normal pregnancy produce a compensated maternal respiratory alkalosis because of increased minute ventilation followed by a reduction in serum bicarbonate. The decrease in serum bicarbonate contributes to a reduction in the overall buffering capacity to handle the acidosis precipitated with DKA.[3,13,16]

Although DKA does not have any pathognomonic features, there are several classic clinical findings that should raise a high level of suspicion to the provider. Patients generally present with abdominal pain, malaise, persistent vomiting, polydypsia, hyperventilation, tachycardia, dehydration, and polyuria. Because of the large burden of keto acids in the blood, patients may present with the characteristic fruity odor of the breath.

As the level of acidosis increases, the patient will often have altered mental status and sometimes present completely obtunded. The diagnosis is confirmed with documentation of hyperglycemia, acidosis, and ketonuria. Other laboratory findings include anion gap, ketonemia, renal dysfunction, as well as possible electrolyte abnormalities.[13,16]

Typically the patient presents with levels of serum glucose >300 mg/dL; however, this threshold is much lower in pregnancy and DKA can occur with levels <200 mg/dL.[14]

Precipitating factors for diabetic ketoacidosis include emesis, infection, previously undiagnosed diabetes, β-sympathomimetic tocolytic agents, corticosteroids, poor compliance, pump malfunctions, and medical errors. Retrospective studies have indicated that emesis, poor compliance, infection, the use of β-sympathomimetics, and medical errors accounted for 80% of the cases of DKA.[17,18] Although β-sympathomimetics (terbutaline) are not used routinely for prolonged (>48 hours) tocolysis due to the Food and Drug Administration safety communication in 2011 warning of the potential for serious maternal heart problems and death, it is important to remember that they should be used very cautiously, if ever, for patients with diabetes.[3]

Maternal DKA presents a significant risk to overall fetal well-being. The mechanism by which maternal DKA affects the fetus is not clearly understood; however, it appears to be related to several factors. Maternal hypovolemia decreases uterine blood flow and keto acids readily cross the placenta, which can decrease tissue perfusion and reduce oxygenation in the fetus. In addition, these keto acids can dissociate into anions and result in fetal metabolic acidosis.[16] The fetus has a limited ability to buffer significant acidemia, and therefore, is quite sensitive to maternal acidosis.

This often results in a fetal heart tracing that may include a nonreactive nonstress test, decreased variability, or late decelerations. The National Institute of Child Health and Human Development category II and III heart tracings are not unusual in a setting of maternal DKA. Interpretation can be difficult considering the high false-positive rates inherent in fetal monitoring. However, it is likely that maternal acidosis, hyperglycemia, and hypovolemia all contribute to a potential threat to fetal well-being.[13] Efforts to correct the maternal acidosis is key to improving the underlying fetal status. It is important to exhaust all attempts to correct the underlying maternal abnormalities before intervening for the fetus.[14,16]

DKA is considered a medical emergency and consultation with Maternal-Fetal Medicine, Neonatology, and Critical Care specialists should occur as soon as possible. In addition, strong consideration should be made for admission to an intensive care unit. After a detailed history and physical examination, intravenous access should be obtained and an indwelling urinary catheter should be placed. Fluid balance and vital signs need to be carefully monitored and documented.

Basic laboratory work, including a complete metabolic panel with magnesium and phosphorous, complete blood count with differential, urinalysis, fingerstick blood glucose, arterial blood gas, and serum ketones should be collected. Additional testing (urine culture, blood culture, chest radiograph, and so on) should be performed based on clinical suspicion and any potential underlying processes. Initially, urine/serum ketones, electrolytes, and maternal acid/base status should be monitored every 2 hours until ketosis and acidosis are resolved. Blood sugars should be collected hourly during this time to titrate appropriate insulin doses.[3,13,16,19,20]

Once viability is confirmed, fetal monitoring should be initiated. As noted, the fetal heart tracing will likely appear concerning during the initial insult. Maternal oxygen supplementation and favorable maternal positioning should be used to increase blood flow to the fetus and improve oxygenation. Adequate hydration and correction of acid/base derangements must be started. Delivery should be postponed until after the maternal metabolic condition is stabilized, as this will usually correct the fetal heart tracing abnormality. There are exceptions, including intractable bradycardia or persistent category III tracings.

Fig. 4 illustrates the goals of treatment of any patient with DKA: rehydration, reduction of hyperglycemia, correction of acid-base and electrolyte imbalance, while searching for and treating the underlying cause.[3,13,16,19,20]

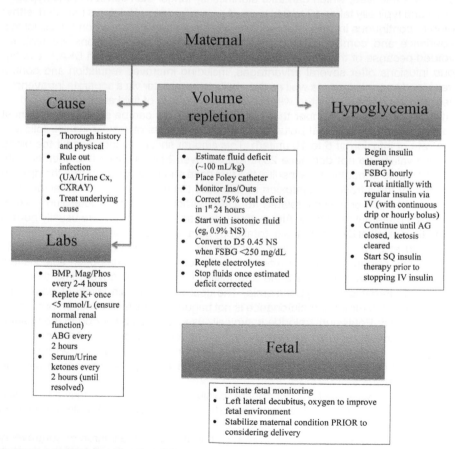

Fig. 4. Treatment algorithm for DKA.

The fluid deficit leading to the profound intravascular depletion is estimated at 100 mL/kg of total body weight and is typically 4 to 10 L.[15] Initially, aggressive intravenous replacement with isotonic normal saline should commence with the goal of replacing approximately 75% of the overall deficit within the first 24 hours. Hypotonic fluids (eg, lactated Ringer and 0.45% saline) should be avoided initially because they can cause a rapid decline in plasma osmolarity, leading to cerebral edema. Blood glucose values should be monitored hourly because they will decrease with initial hydration alone. Once the serum glucose reaches <250 mg/dL, fluids should be switched to D5–0.45% normal saline. It is important to monitor urinary output and fluids should not be stopped until the entire calculated deficit is replaced.

Intravenous insulin administration should be undertaken immediately in DKA to inhibit the lipolysis and ketogenesis associated with increased levels of serum glucose. One efficient way to correct serum glucose is an intravenous insulin drip. Regular insulin of 1 unit per milliliter in 100 mL 0.9% NaCl solution is prepared by the pharmacy and the rate of infusion is calculated based on the level of blood glucose and entered into the pump. There are several available calculators and many institutions have protocols for adjusting insulin dosage. The initial blood glucose target is 150 to 200 mg/dL to avoid rapid correction and resulting complications.

It is important to continue the insulin infusion until the anion gap is closed and acidosis is resolved, which can take significantly longer than correcting the hypoglycemia and typically takes 12 to 24 hours. If an insulin drip calculator is not used, either bolus or continuous infusion approaches can be used safely based on the clinician's experience and comfort. Subcutaneous and intramuscular injections are typically avoided because of the slower onset of action, which is worsened in DKA.[13] Continuous infusions offer several advantages, including improved regulation and control over blood sugar values, as well as the ability to administer via a separate intravenous line and thus can be adjusted without affecting the rate of fluid administration.

It is important to remember that insulin requirements can be significant and most protocols suggest an initial bolus dose of 10 to 20 units of regular insulin, followed by a rate of infusion of 5 to 10 units/h. This amount should be increased if the blood glucose values do not decrease 25% to 20% over 2 hours. Once it is deemed safe to transition to subcutaneous insulin, the first dose should be given before the discontinuation of the intravenous infusion to decrease the risk of recurrent ketoacidosis.

Electrolyte abnormalities related to DKA particularly involve potassium, which increases maternal morbidity. Although levels of serum potassium are usually normal at the time of initial DKA diagnosis, total body potassium is low and the actual deficit is estimated at 5 to 10 meq/kg and replacement should begin after fluid and insulin therapy has begun, as well as after adequate renal function has been established. Potassium is excreted in the urine and insulin treatment will drive it into the cells, resulting in intravascular hypokalemia. The goal is to maintain levels of potassium between 4 and 5 mmol/L; maintenance is not begun until the level of serum potassium drops below 5. Potassium chloride is typically used and can be added to the maintenance IV fluids or repleted separately with an expected increase of 0.1 mmol/L per 10 meq replacement. Renal function should be monitored and levels of serum potassium should be checked every 2 to 4 hours. Significant hypokalemia can precipitate a cardiac arrhythmia.

Other electrolytes, such as phosphate, calcium, and magnesium, may also be low and should be replaced as well, although studies have not shown a direct benefit in DKA.

Replacement of levels of low serum bicarbonate remains a source of controversy and replacement is generally agreed on if the patient's pH is <7.0. Some studies have shown that routine replacement of low serum levels of bicarbonate have not proven beneficial in DKA and may cause unnecessary maternal and fetal complications. Replacement can delay the correction of keto acids in the maternal bloodstream and, if corrected too rapidly, elevate fetal PCO_2, impairing fetal ability to maintain adequate O_2 transfer.[3,20]

HYPOGLYCEMIA

Hypoglycemia is an uncommon, although potentially dangerous, complication of pregnancy. As the control of blood glucose in pregnancy has been tightened, many diabetics patients, especially type I, are at risk for hypoglycemia. Although hypoglycemia is not strongly associated with maternal mortality—like hyperglycemia (DKA), prolonged severe hypoglycemia can result in a hypoglycemic coma or seizures.[14]

Hypoglycemia is defined as serum glucose <60 mg/dL. The incidence, although difficult to estimate, has been reported in approximately 35% of diabetic patients with the vast majority occurring in type I diabetics. Other risk factors include prior history of hypoglycemia and poor compliance.

The response to hypoglycemia typically consists of the release of counterregulatory hormones to increase serum glucose values. This response is blunted in diabetic pregnant patients who typically maintain tight control, which can also result in the inability of the patient to perceive the "low," leading to worsening hypoglycemia. Typical symptoms including tremors and sweating may only manifest at very low levels. Unless very profound hypoglycemia exists, there are few significant maternal hemodynamic or fetal effects.[14]

Episodes are treated with rapid glucose replacement in the form of juice, a snack, or glucose tablets. Simple carbohydrates work quickly and are preferred over complex carbohydrates and proteins. Glucagon should be administered if the patient is unable to swallow. Isolated episodes do not typically warrant hospital admission.

An effort should be made to identify the underlying cause of hypoglycemia in affected patients. Adjustment of maternal insulin therapy, dietary evaluation, and/or the initiation of a snack should be considered. Those patients who have recurrent episodes of hypoglycemia despite conventional measures should undergo a more thorough workup. Dietary and lifestyle habits should be reviewed, and measurement of serum C-peptide and potential referral to Endocrinology or Maternal-Fetal Medicine specialists should be considered. Driving and activity precautions need to be discussed with the patient and their families. Clinicians should consider the excess administration of exogenous insulin as a causative factor and a psychiatric evaluation may be appropriate.

Animal studies have shown an increase in neural tube defects and growth reduction, although teratogenic effects have not been proven in human fetuses. There was concern in some studies associating maternal hypoglycemia with fetal heart rate abnormalities, although this has not been substantiated in subsequent trials.[14]

DIABETES INSIPIDUS

Diabetes insipidus (DI) is a rare condition of polydipsia and polyuria resulting from an inability to concentrate urine. Despite the name, it is physiologically unrelated to diabetes mellitus. It may result from decreased production of antidiuretic hormone (ADH) or decreased sensitivity to ADH in the kidney. Decreased production of ADH in the hypothalamus has typically been described as central DI, but there is a gestational variant that results from increased destruction of ADH in the placenta.

The presentation of DI often mimics uncontrolled diabetes, with severe thirst, frequent urination, nocturia, and fatigue. Unlike diabetes, patients with DI will have hypo-osmolar urine, usually <200 mOsm/kg. Differentiating central from renal DI may require a water deprivation test, level of plasma ADH, or both.

Treatment of DI is usually desmopressin, or DDAVP, which is an ADH analog. Available in nasal spray, IV, and oral forms, it is effective and well tolerated. The typical intranasal dose is 20 to 30 ug once or twice per day. Renal DI may be resistant to this treatment. Pregnancy-related DI usually responds to DDAVP and would be expected to improve postpartum. Cases of associated uterine atony and pre-eclampsia have been reported, but most patients do well in pregnancy.[21]

HYPOPARATHYROIDISM

Hypoparathyroidism is a condition characterized by severe hypocalcemia, which manifests with muscle spasms, tetany, and changes in mental status. Severe cases may progress to seizures, myocardial infarction, and even death.[22] Parathyroid hormone is a significant determinate of calcium homeostasis, influencing the efflux of calcium from bone and the absorption of calcium from the intestinal tract and the kidneys.

The most common cause of hypoparathyroidism is inadvertent destruction of the 4 glands, which are tucked behind the thyroid. Hypoparathyroidism is most likely to occur during partial or complete thyroidectomy. External radiation and even radionuclear ablation can be less common causes. Autoimmunity accounts for a minority of cases, which results in infiltration and destruction of the gland, similar to Hashimoto thyroiditis. Rarely, hypoparathyroidism can be associated with other medical conditions, such as malignancy, Wilson disease, and DiGeorge syndrome.

The diagnosis is usually made by physical evidence of generalized muscle spasms, along with low levels of serum total and ionized calcium. Paresthesias and mental status changes may also be observed. Elevated serum phosphate and decreased or absent parathyroid hormone (PTH) and calcitriol are also common findings. Electrocardiogram findings of bradycardia or prolonged QT segments can indicate pending cardiac failure.

The mainstay of treatment is intravenous calcium replacement, either calcium gluconate or elemental calcium. Elemental calcium can be given 1 to 2 mg/kg/h as an infusion. Supportive care, careful fetal monitoring, and specific treatment of seizures or cardiac symptoms are also required. Long-term therapy consists of increased calcium intake from diet and supplementation, as well as Vitamin D supplementation to mimic the actions of PTH.

Neonatal hyperparathyroidism has been described in response to maternal hypoparathyroidism.[23] Neonatal hyperparathyroidism may result in fetal growth restriction and skeletal fractures. Infant deaths have been reported as a result. Pediatricians and neonatologists should be mindful of this potential serious sequelae.

HYPERPARATHYROIDISM

Hyperparathyroidism is a condition of increased PTH and hypercalcemia.[22] It is relatively rare in pregnancy. Most patients are asymptomatic for significant periods of time. Once it becomes severe or poorly controlled, common symptoms include kidney stones, hypertension, gastrointestinal complaints, mental status changes, and bone pain.[24] Long-standing hyperparathyroidism may result in fractures or curvature of bone. Mortality in pregnancy has been reported.[24]

Most commonly a single hyperfunctioning adenoma is the cause of the excess PTH. Less often, all 4 glands may undergo hyperplasia. The source of PTH may be the glands themselves or can be from an exogenous source.

Significant elevations of PTH and serum calcium, along with systemic symptoms, will clinch the diagnosis. Maternal adaptations to pregnancy may mask the total serum calcium increases. Thyroid storm, milk-alkali syndrome, and malignancy may be confused with hyperparathyroidism.

The definitive treatment is surgery, which is attempted to be as minimally invasive as possible.[24] Preoperative imaging may be useful in localizing the problem areas and focusing the surgical effort. The second trimester is the ideal time for most surgeries, but it could be performed almost any time in pregnancy. The prognosis after surgery is good, with well over 90% of patients experiencing a resolution of symptoms.

Acute hypercalcemia is a medical emergency and requires medical management as well. Vigorous hydration and diuretic therapy are mainstays of treatment, along with IV phosphates and Calcitonin to decrease bone resorption. **Box 2** summarizes treatment options and doses (see **Box 2**).

PHEOCHROMOCYTOMA

Pheochromocytoma is a tumor of the adrenal medulla that secretes significant amounts of catecholamine. Most of these tumors are benign; however, systemic side effects of the catecholamines can lead to maternal mortality. Pheochromocytomas have also been reported in other sites of the body besides the adrenal gland and these ectopic tumors have a higher incidence of malignant potential.

Patients often present with uncontrollable or rapidly progressive hypertension, which is an effect from significant α-adrenergic and β-adrenergic stimulation. The hypertension may be labile and take significant swings over a 24-hour period. Other symptoms include headache, chest pain, restlessness, seizures, and cardiovascular collapse. The symptoms and signs can sometimes be confused with patients experiencing HELLP syndrome or hypertensive crisis with chronic hypertension in pregnancy.

The diagnosis can be made by plasma and urine assessments of catecholamines and metanephrines. Values are not substantially altered by the maternal adaptations of pregnancy. Once pheochromocytoma is suspected on laboratory analysis, it may be confirmed by imaging studies, either magnetic resonance imaging or computed tomography.

Definitive treatment is surgical removal of the tumor. The timing and type of surgery are a complex decision, one made best with multidisciplinary consultation. Medical management, using α-blockade alpha and β-blockade have been described.[25] Medical management with α-blockade alpha and β-blockade is an attractive option for poor surgical candidates, unknown location of the tumor, and diagnosis between 24 and 32 weeks of pregnancy.

ADDISON'S DISEASE (ADRENAL INSUFFICIENCY)

Adrenal insufficiency is a rare but potentially dangerous condition in pregnancy. Historically it has carried a significant risk of maternal mortality and fetal morbidity, including preterm delivery.[26,27] The most common causes of adrenal failure include auto-immune destruction, hemorrhage, and malignancy. The onset may be acute or gradual. Symptoms of abdominal pain, nausea, anorexia, weakness, and confusion may be present, but are nonspecific. Diagnosis may be made with an adrenocorticotropic hormone

(ACTH) stimulation test, although rapid diagnosis can sometimes be made with serum cortisol and ACTH.

Replacement of glucocorticoids is the mainstay of treatment.[28] In acute situations, 100 mg cortisol IV given every 8 to 12 hours can be life-saving. Definitive diagnosis via ACTH stimulation test may be delayed if clinical suspicion is high. Chronic insufficiency may be treated with lower dose oral replacement. Stress dosing is required for situations of stress, such as surgery or delivery.

REFERENCES

1. Tietgens ST, Leinung MC. Thyroid Storm. Med Clin North Am 1995;79:169–84.
2. Goldberg PA. Critical issues in endocrinology. Clin Chest Med 2003;24:583–606.
3. Parker JA, Conway DL. Diabetic ketoacidosis in pregnancy. Obstet Gynecol Clin North Am 2007;34:533–43.
4. Nayak B, Burman K. Thyrotoxicosis and thyroid storm. Endocrinol Metab Clin North Am 2006;35:663–86.
5. Burch HB, Wartofsky L. Thyroid storm. Endocrinol Metab Clin North Am 1993;22: 263–77.
6. Delport EF. A thyroid-related endocrine emergency in pregnancy. JEMDSA 2009; 14(2):99–201.
7. Rashid M, Rashid MH. Obstetric management of thyroid disease. Obstet Gynecol Surv 2007;62(10):680–8.
8. Bahn RS, Burch H, Copper D, et al. Hyperthyroidism and other causes of thyrotoxicosis: management guidelines of the ATA and the AACE. Endocr Pract 2011; 17(3):456–520.
9. Gianantonio E, Schaefer C, Mastroiacovo P. Adverse fetal effects of prenatal methimazole exposure. Teratology 2001;64(5):262–6.
10. Vyas AA, Vyas P, Fillipon NP, et al. Successful treatment of thyroid storm with plasmaphoresis in a patient with MMI-induced agranulocytosis. Endocr Pract 2010;16(4):673–6.
11. Turhan NO, Kockar M, Inegol I. Myxedematous coma in a laboring woman suggested a pre-eclamptic coma: a case report. Acta Obstet Gynecol Scand 2004;83(11):1089–91.
12. Dutta P, Bhansali A, Mansoodi S, et al. Predictors of outcome in myxedema coma: a study from a tertiary care center. Crit Care 2008;12:R1, 1–8.
13. Abdu TA, Barton DM, Baskar V, et al. Diabetic ketoacidosis on pregnancy. Postgrad Med J 2003;79(934):454.
14. Whiteman VE, Homko CJ, Reece EA. Management of hypoglycemia and diabetic ketoacidosis in pregnancy. Obstet Gynecol Clin North Am 1996;23(1):88–107.
15. Chauhan SP, Perry KG, McLaughlin BN, et al. Diabetic ketoacidosis complicating pregnancy. J Perinatol 1996;16(1):173–5.
16. Carroll M, Yeomans ER. Diabetic ketoacidosis in pregnancy. Crit Care Med 2005; 33:S347–53.
17. Rogers BD, Rogers DE. Clinical variable associated with diabetic ketoacidosis during pregnancy. J Reprod Med 1991;36:797–800.
18. Montoro MN, Myers VP, Mestman JH, et al. Outcome of pregnancy in diabetic ketoacidosis. Am J Perinatol 1993;10:17–20.
19. Ramin K. Diabetic ketoacidosis in pregnancy. Obstet Gynecol Clin North Am 1999;26(3):481–8.
20. Foley MR, Strong TH, Garite TJ. Obstetric intensive care manual. 2nd edition. New York: McGraw Hill Publishers; 2004.

21. Hendricks CH. The neurohypophysis in pregnancy. Obstet Gynecol Surv 1954;9: 323.
22. Mestman JH. Parathyroid disorders of pregnancy. Semin Perinatol 1998;22:485.
23. Loughead JL, Mughal Z, Mimouni F, et al. Spectrum and natural history of congenital hyperparathyroidism secondary to maternal hypocalcemia. Am J Perinatol 1990;7:350.
24. Kristofferson A, Dahlgren S, Lithner F, et al. Primary hyperparathyroidism and pregnancy. Surgery 1985;97:326.
25. Lyons CW, Colmorgen GC. Medical management of pheochromocytoma. Obstet Gynecol 1988;72:450.
26. Brent F. Addison's disease and pregnancy. Am J Surg 1950;79:645.
27. Bjornsdottir S, Cnattingius S, Brandt L. Addison's disease in women is a risk factor for an adverse pregnancy outcome. J Clin Endocrinol Metab 2010;95(12): 5249–57.
28. Adonakis G, Georgopoulus NA, Michail G, et al. Successful pregnancy outcome in a patient with Addison's disease. Gynecol Endocrinol 2005;21(2):90–2.

Placenta Accreta, Increta, and Percreta

Alison C. Wortman, MD*, James M. Alexander, MD

KEYWORDS

- Placenta • Accreta • Increta • Percreta • Pregnancy • Abnormal • Placentation
- Hemorrhage

KEY POINTS

- Women at highest risk for placenta accreta have a history of a prior cesarean delivery with the current pregnancy complicated by placenta previa as well as placental implantation over the prior uterine scar.
- Gray-scale ultrasound has 77% to 86% sensitivity and 96% to 98% specificity for diagnosis of placenta accreta.
- Delivery timing should be individualized but generally planned around 34 to 35 weeks estimated gestational age.
- Planned cesarean hysterectomy with no attempt at placental delivery is standard management.
- Alternative approaches, such as leaving the placenta in situ without hysterectomy, have increased risks and should be reserved for individualized patients.

INTRODUCTION

The first mention of placenta accreta was in the late 1500s by Plater, who tells of a noble lady in 88 AD who delivered, had a retained placenta, and died; on autopsy, the placenta was found to be firmly adhered around the internal os.[1] Because placenta accreta was so rare before the 1970s, the reported incidence varied, but Breen and colleagues[2] looked at the average of reports from 1871 to 1972 and found it to be 1 in 7000 deliveries. Read and colleagues[3] alarmingly reported an increasing rate of 1 in 4027 deliveries in the 1970s, but the most recent data from 1982 to 2002 show the current incidence of placenta accreta to be a staggering 1 in 533 deliveries.[4,5] This increase is likely secondary to the rising rate of cesarean delivery in the United States, from 5% of all deliveries in 1970 climbing to 32.8% in 2010 (**Fig. 1**).[6,7] Placenta

Funding Sources: None.
Conflict of Interest: None.
Department of Maternal Fetal Medicine, University of Texas Southwestern Medical Center, 5323 Harry Hines Boulevard, Dallas, TX 75390, USA
* Corresponding author.
E-mail address: Alison.Wortman@UTSouthwestern.edu

Obstet Gynecol Clin N Am 40 (2013) 137–154
http://dx.doi.org/10.1016/j.ogc.2012.12.002
0889-8545/13/$ – see front matter Published by Elsevier Inc.

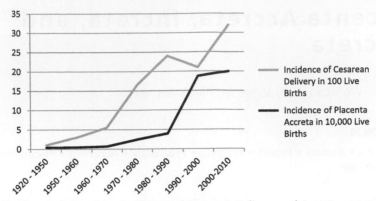

Fig. 1. Graph comparing rising incidence of Cesarean Delivery and Accreta.

accreta is well known to cause significant increased maternal and neonatal morbidity and mortality, and with its increasing occurrence, every obstetrician must be familiar with the most current diagnostic and treatment options.

DEFINITIONS

Placenta accreta is a generalized term used when an abnormal, firmly adherent placenta implants with some degree of invasion into the uterus. It occurs as a consequence of partial or complete absence of the deciduas basalis and defective formation of the Nitabuch (fibrinoid) layer. The anomalous attachment can be described based on the number of lobules involved:

- *Total placenta accreta*: involves all lobules
- *Partial placenta accreta*: involves at least 2 but not all of the lobules
- *Focal placenta accreta*: involves only a single lobule, either a portion or the entire lobule

The 3 classifications of adherent placentas are based on the degree of invasion and include the following:

- *Accreta*: placental villi are attached to the myometrium
- *Increta*: invasion of the placental villi into the myometrium (**Fig. 2**)
- *Percreta*: placenta villa fully penetrate the myometrium, including cases breaching the serosa and invading surrounding structures, such as the bladder, broad ligament, or sigmoid colon[8]

RISK FACTORS

Women at highest risk for placenta accreta have myometrial damage from a previous cesarean delivery and a subsequent pregnancy with placenta previa as well as implantation of the placenta over the prior uterine scar. The risk for placenta accreta in a patient with placenta previa and prior cesarean delivery increases with number of previous cesarean deliveries. Silver and colleagues[9] reported the risk for the first, second, third, fourth, and fifth or greater cesarean delivery to be 3.3%, 11%, 40%, 61%, and 67%. Previous cesarean delivery alone, without previa, is also an independent risk factor for accreta with increasing incidence associated with increasing number of cesareans; 0.2% for the first, 2.1% with the fourth, and up to 6.7% with

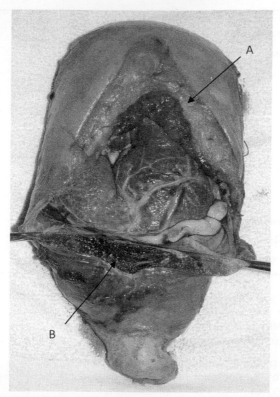

Fig. 2. Placenta increta showing (*A*) normal uterine wall and (*B*) uterine wall with placental invasion to the myometrium. (*Photograph courtesy of* Dr Barbara Hoffman, Dallas, TX.)

the sixth or greater. In addition, placenta previa alone without previous uterine surgery is associated with a 1% to 4% risk of accreta.[4,9] Advanced maternal age is also a reported independent risk factor for accreta with the risk increasing for every year beyond 20 years of age.[5] Additional risk factors include uterine surgery, such as myomectomy, endometrial ablation, and dilation and curettage (**Box 1**).[4,5,9–12]

DIAGNOSIS

Prenatal diagnosis and knowledge of the extent of placental invasion are instrumental in optimizing patient outcomes in placenta accreta. Foreknowledge allows referral to a tertiary care center, multidisciplinary approach when necessary, and meticulous planning. The mainstay of prenatal diagnosis for abnormal placentation remains duplex ultrasonography with magnetic resonance imaging (MRI) being used only as an adjunct in indeterminate cases. An ultrasound or MRI diagnosis of placenta accreta predicts the need for hysterectomy with a sensitivity of 78%, 67%, and a specificity of 67%, 50%, respectively.[13]

Ultrasound

In general, gray-scale ultrasonography predicts abnormal placentation with a sensitivity of 77% to 86%, specificity 96% to 98%, positive predictive value 63% to 88%, and negative predictive value 95% to 98%.[14–16] With 3-dimensional power Doppler, visualizing numerous coherent vessels on the basal view has been reported

---

Box 1
Risk factors for placenta accreta

- Both previous cesarean delivery and placenta previa
- Previous cesarean delivery
- Placenta previa
- Advanced maternal age
- Previous uterine surgery
  - Myomectomy
  - Metroplasty
- Severe endometrial damage
  - Ashermans
  - Submucosal fibroid
- Endometrial ablation
- Uterine artery embolization

---

to have a sensitivity of 97% and a specificity of 92%.[17] The additional use of color flow Doppler or power flow Doppler does not significantly approve diagnostic sensitivity over gray-scale ultrasonography alone.[14]

Ultrasonographic findings suggestive of placenta accreta (**Fig. 3**) are as follows:

- Presence of multiple placenta lacunae[15,16] (sensitivity 93%)
- Interruption of the posterior bladder wall-uterine interface[14–16] (sensitivity 20%, specificity 100%)
- Obliteration of the clear space between the uterus and placenta[14–16] (sensitivity 80%, positive predictive value 6%)
- Hypervascularity of the adjacent bladder wall[14,16]
- Smallest myometrial thickness <1 mm[18]

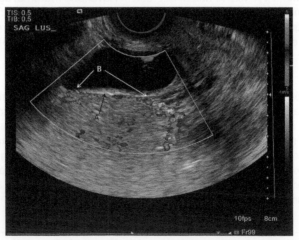

Fig. 3. 34 wk ultrasound of placenta increta pictured at time of surgery in Figure 2 showing (*A*) attenuation of the retroplacental myometrium, with (*B*) prominent retroplacental vessels that bridge to the uterine serosa. This image is from the same patient whose uterus is shown after planned cesarean hysterectomy in the other images.

Assessment of depth of myometrial invasion has not been studied as much as the accuracy of general diagnosis of accreta but useful criteria for depth of invasion include the following[19]:

- Vessels extending from the placenta to the bladder
- Vessels crossing the interruption of the placental-tissue interface (the more complex the vascular pattern in the myometrium the deeper the invasion)

Magnetic Resonance Imaging

Most investigators have found similar diagnostic accuracy between MRI and ultrasonography but because of the higher cost of MRI and the level of expertise required for proper interpretation, it is usually only recommended for ambiguous cases. Less data have been reported on the accuracy of MRI in predicting placenta accreta but the sensitivity ranges from 78% to 88% and the specificity ranges from 67% to 100%. The most valuable features of placenta accreta on MRI are the following[13,16,20]:

- Dark intraplacental bands on T2-weighted sequences
- Uterine bulging
- Heterogeneous signal intensity within the placenta

An Argentinean prospective study found 100% prediction of parametrial invasion with MRI but they used gross diagnosis in the operating room and not histology for final placental topography and level of invasion. They also noted that slice thickness and the use of image filters can affect the MRI's diagnostic error with slice thickeners less than 7 mm with an increase in false positives and mid-image and high-image filters helping to eliminate artifact created by neoformation vessels but leading to an underestimation of the degree of invasion.[21] Although the use of gandolinium did not alter the sensitivity of diagnosing accreta, gandolinium-enhanced images did define the location of the outer surface of the placenta relative to the myometrium.[16]

The use of gadolinium in pregnancy continues to be controversial. Gadolinium is known to cross the placenta to the fetus in rabbits and concentrations in the placenta and fetal kidneys were high enough for imaging and possibly fetal toxicity.[22] There is no evidence of teratogenicity with gadolinium use in rats, rabbits, and monkeys even when given repeatedly during organogenesis at doses 25 times (monkeys) and 100 times (rats, rabbits) the diagnostic dose in humans, and it is quickly cleared from fetal circulation in rats.[23,24] However, at 2.5 times the human dose in rats and 7.5 to 12.5 times the human dosage in rabbits, gadolinium exposure was associated with minor developmental delay.[22] Gandolinium exposure has also been reported to increase the risk of nephrogenic systemic fibrosis, a rare, potentially lethal, systemic fibrotic disorder, in patients with significantly impaired renal function.[25] It is not known if nephrogenic systemic fibrosis could also be potentiated in the fetus after gadolinium exposure. The American College of Radiology recommends that MRI be used in pregnancy only if the diagnostic information cannot be obtained with nonionizing means, such as ultrasonography, and the data are needed to guide the care of the mother or fetus during the current pregnancy. They further specify that MRI contrast agents should not be used routinely in pregnancy and their use is only justified with "overwhelming potential benefit to the patient or fetus."[26] In ambiguous cases where MRI may be the key to prenatal diagnosis of placenta accreta, the benefits of proper planning and optimizing maternal outcomes may outweigh the possible fetal risks.

MANAGEMENT

The standard of care for suspected placenta accreta is planned cesarean hysterectomy with the placenta left in situ. Uterine-sparing options have been reported, but recognizing that morbidity can be high and further intervention will often be necessary, these options should be reserved for individualized patients. Even with a planned cesarean hysterectomy, certain management modalities and techniques can aid in improving outcomes.

Preparation for Delivery

Referral to a tertiary care center and a multidisciplinary approach have been shown to improve patient outcomes.[27] The disciplines involved should include maternal-fetal medicine, anesthesiology, pathology for blood banking, neonatology, and gynecologic oncology. Urology, vascular surgery, and interventional radiology may also be useful teams to include depending on the level of placental invasion and anatomy involved.[28] The hospital where the patient is delivered must have an adequate blood bank that can support massive transfusion if required at time of delivery.

Routine supplementation with iron and folic acid can aid in anemia prevention preoperatively. A hematocrit of greater than 30 is a reasonable goal.[29] Some even advocate the use of erythropoietin to achieve this goal. Erythropoietin is made by the kidneys and increases red blood cell mass by stimulating the bone marrow. Its main use is for anemia associated with renal failure but has been given in pregnancy for anemia without renal disease.[30,31] It has been shown to decrease the need for transfusion as well as increase the level of hemoglobin and erythrocyte count in normal preoperative patients undergoing hip replacement.[32] This effect is likely due to an erythroid progenitor amplification followed by a gradual increase of erythroblasts.[33] The patient must have normal iron stores or be supplemented with iron.[30,34] Although not yet reported in pregnant patients who have received erythropoietin, it can have side effects such as hypertension, a flu-like syndrome, conjunctival inflammation, and rare, more serious side effects, such as seizure and thrombotic events.[34,35] It does not seem to pose a major risk to the fetus and does not cross the placenta.[35]

Most patients who undergo a cesarean hysterectomy will need a blood transfusion; therefore, ensuring that the patient does not have any rare alloantibodies before delivery is also important.

Delivery Timing

The July 2012 American College of Obstetrics and Gynecology committee opinion on placenta accreta stated that delivery timing for placenta accreta must be individualized. Obstetricians must perform thorough counseling to include discussion of the high potential for hysterectomy, profuse hemorrhage, probable transfusion, increased complications, and possible maternal death.[36] Compared to emergent peripartum hysterectomy, planned obstetric hysterectomy has been shown to have decreased intraoperative blood loss, less intraoperative hypotension, and decreased chance of requiring a blood transfusion when compared with emergent peripartum hysterectomy.[37] The patient and obstetrician must weigh the risks of neonatal prematurity and the benefit of a planned delivery before the onset of labor. Hemorrhage from labor and cervical dilation must be avoided if possible, especially in the setting of a placenta accreta with previa. Patients with placenta previa and a cervical length of 30 mm or less at 32 weeks have been found to have an increased risk of hemorrhage, uterine activity, and preterm birth.[38]

Numerous approaches exist regarding the appropriate gestational age for delivery. A 2010 decision analysis tree suggested that the preferred strategy was delivery at

34 weeks without amniocentesis for placenta previa with suspected accreta. The authors made several assumptions about lifetime affects of certain outcomes, such as maternal intensive care unit admission, that may have skewed their results. They also reported that amniocentesis for fetal lung maturity did not affect outcomes at any gestational age.[39] An expert opinion in 2010 recommended delivery for uncomplicated previa at 36 to 37 weeks estimated gestational age and 34 to 35 weeks for suspected placental invasion.[40] According to a recent survey of 508 members of Society for Maternal Fetal Medicine, many maternal-fetal medicine practitioners perform amniocentesis for fetal lung maturity before delivery (46.8%), which they most commonly schedule at 36 weeks (48.4%).[41] Although a planned cesarean hysterectomy should be the goal, an emergency contingency plan should also be outlined that should include institutional protocols for massive transfusion and how to contact each member of the multidisciplinary care team afterhours.

In summary, each patient must be evaluated and an individualized delivery plan must be formed based on placental location, extent of invasion, cervical length, clinical course in the pregnancy, and capabilities of the delivering facility and care team.

Anesthesia

With increased experience and modifications of technique, neuraxial anesthesia has become more common in deliveries involving placenta accreta.[42] Continuous epidural anesthesia and combined spinal-epidural anesthesia are both viable options with a reported rate of conversion to general anesthesia of about 28% to 29% when regional anesthesia was first used.[42,43] Difficulty of the maternal airway, degree of placental invasion, expected amount of hemorrhage, length of surgical time, and degree of dissection should all be considered for anesthesia management. If a difficult airway,[42] extensive dissection, prolonged operating time, and massive hemorrhage are anticipated, general anesthesia is commonly recommended.[43]

Resuscitation

When a large blood loss is anticipated, several techniques can be used to decrease the chance of allogenic transfusion:

- Autologous blood donation/transfusion
- Acute normovolemic hemodilution
- Intraoperative cell salvage
- Hemostatic resuscitation

Autologous blood donations in pregnancy can safely be performed after 30 weeks of gestation but require a starting hematocrit of 34 and at least 2 weeks of recovery before surgery.[44] The cost and improbability that patients in advanced pregnancy with abnormal placentation will be able to make adequate autologous donations to avoid homologous transfusion hinder its usefulness in the average patient with placenta accreta, but patients with rare antibodies may be candidates for autologous blood donations.

Acute normovolemic hemodilution (ANH) is begun in the operating room before the start of surgery. Two to 3 units of whole blood are collected from the patient and replaced by colloid/crystalloid to maintain normovolemia. The remaining intravascular blood has a lower number of red cells to lose during surgery and autologous fresh whole blood with the starting red blood cell concentration and all the active clotting factors as well as functional platelets can been transfused back after hemostasis is secured. The patient must have an initial hemoglobin of at least 10 g/dL, no history of cardiac disease, and a predicted blood loss of at least 20% of the patient's blood volume. The collected blood may be stored at room temperature for up to 6 hours. Although autologous blood donation and transfusion are not acceptable to Jehovah's Witnesses, as long as the collection bag remains connected to the central venous line at all times (no circuit disconnections), ANH is acceptable to most Jehovah's Witnesses. In general, evidence suggests that ANH alone does not spare significant quantities of allogenic blood but may be useful for an estimated blood loss of up to 2000 mL.[45]

Intraoperative cell salvage or cell saver usage has also been described as an option in obstetrics. Blood is aspirated from the surgical field through heparinized tubing and filtered into a collecting reservoir. The cells are separated, centrifuged, and washed to remove particles such as circulating fibrin, debris, plasma, platelets, microaggregates, complement, circulating procoagulants, and most of the heparin. Up to 250 mL of packed red blood cells with a hematocrit of 50 to 80 can be returned to the patient within 3 minutes of aspiration.[45] Although there is clearance of humoral material, maternal-fetal blood cells remain in postprocessed blood.[46] Some theoretical concerns exist about increasing the risk of amniotic fluid embolism and Rhesus isoimmunization with cell salvage use in obstetrics, but amniotic fluid embolism has never been documented in over 400 published cases and Rhesus isoimmunization can be avoided as long as Rh-negative patients receive the appropriate amount of anti-D immunoglobulin, according to their Kleihauer Betke stain.[45] However, isoimmunization against other antigens, such as Kidd, Kell, or Duffy, is also possible.[46] This technique does require preplanning and the allocation of personnel trained in its use for the delivery. It has been reported as an effective option when severe obstetric hemorrhage is predicted.[45,46]

In the late 1990s, patients with massive hemorrhage were resuscitated with large volumes of crystalloid and packed red blood cells (PRBCs). Other products, such as fresh frozen plasma (FFP), platelets, and cryoprecipitate, were used only as indicated by abnormal hematologic parameters, such as fibrinogen <100 mg/dL, platelets <50,000/mm^3, or abnormal coagulation studies. Not only did this approach fail to prevent coagulopathies in massive hemorrhage but also the liberal use of crystalloid/PRBCs alone creates a dilution of clotting factors or "dilutional coagulopathy." Hypothermia and acidosis can further aggravate the patient's coagulation dysfunction.[47]

Acute traumatic coagulopathy occurs in the setting of severe tissue injury and massive blood loss. The coagulopathy in some cases occurs before dilutional resuscitation. It is partially mediated by the protein C system, whereby activated protein C affects coagulopathy by both inhibiting clot formation and down-regulating the repression of fibrinolysis.[48] The use of whole blood in obstetric hemorrhage has been shown to address possible coagulopathy, decrease the rate of acute tubular necrosis, and reduce the donor exposures.[49] When whole blood is not available, military and civilian data point to improved rates of survival in massive hemorrhage with early administration of FFP and platelets with a 1:1:1 ratio of PRBC:FFP:platelets. Data suggest this may prevent the early development of coagulopathy but some concern exists that survival bias (sicker patients not having enough time to receive thawed FFP) plays a role in these findings and a large prospective trial is currently being performed by the Department of Defense. Aggressive crystalloid resuscitation is avoided not only to prevent hemodilution but also to circumvent clots breaking free after volume expansion and increasing blood pressure. In addition, keeping the systolic blood pressure between 80 and 100 mm Hg may be optimal to limit continuing blood loss.[48]

Recombinant factor VIIa has been shown to limit the amount of blood products transfused in hemorrhage but has not been shown to have a survival benefit. There are no prospective randomized trials in obstetrics but obstetric case reports and series have been published. Recombinant factor VIIa binds to tissue factor and activates the clotting cascade so fibrinogen and clotting factors must be present for it to be effective. There are also valid concerns about thromboembolism associated with its use.[47]

These theories have led to hemostatic resuscitation, which has 3 main concepts:

1. Permissive hypotension
2. 1:1:1 ratio transfusion of PRBC:FFP:platelets
3. Early use of recombinant factor VIIa

Although these concepts were developed for trauma patients, some evidence exists that increased fibrinolytic activity and similar processes also occur in obstetric hemorrhage, and this modern resuscitation technique is often used in massive obstetric hemorrhage.[47]

Interventional Radiology

Therapies in conjunction with interventional radiology, such as internal iliac balloon catheterization or postpartum arterial embolization, have been described with mixed results. Usually preoperative placement of bilateral endovascular internal iliac artery balloons occurs followed by inflation and subsequent occlusion of the bilateral internal iliac arteries after delivery of the infant. Decreased mean blood loss, mean blood volume transfused, and duration of surgery have been reported in some studies but with no difference in mean hemoglobin change or intensive care unit admission.[50] Other reviews report no significant difference in major clinical outcomes when arterial occlusion is used.[51,52] Of note, major complications, such as vascular injury, thrombus formation, and compromised vascular supply to distal extremities, have been reported with these techniques.[53]

Aortic occlusion with a balloon catheter has also been described for temporary control of obstetric hemorrhage. Although there were no complications from the aortic balloon in an Italian study of 18 women and a decreased rate of hysterectomy, estimated blood loss, number of transfused units of PRBCs, postoperative stay, and intensive care unit admissions,[54] an earlier case series had 1 case complicated by aortic rupture.[55]

Surgical Technique

Operation times with placenta accreta are often prolonged so patient positioning is an important detail. If possible, placing the patient in the dorsal lithotomy position with a leftward tilt and hips abducted but with limited hip flexion allows direct estimation of vaginal blood loss during surgery, vaginal and uretheral access for possible vaginal packing or ureteral stent placement/cystoscopy, and an additional space for an assistant to stand. Although most cesarean deliveries are now performed via a Pfannenstiel incision, in the presence of a probable accreta a median or paramedian skin incision (**Fig. 4**) may be preferable for the advantages of improved visibility and superior access to the fundus or even posterior uterine wall for possible alternative hysterotomy sites as well as for hysterectomy.[56]

If the surgery is begun with a Pfannenstiel incision and exposure is not adequate, the best approach is to perform a modified Cherney incision. The rectus muscles should be dissected from the pyramidalis muscles and the anterior rectus sheath followed by transecting the rectus tendons at their insertion into the pubic bone. During closure, the rectus tendons should be reattached to the inferior portion of the rectus sheath, not to the pubic symphysis, to avoid osteomyelitis. Attempting conversion to a Maylard incision or "half-transecting" the rectus abdominis muscles in this circumstance is discouraged because the prior separation of the rectus abdominis muscles and rectus fascia prevents appropriate healing of the transected muscles.[57]

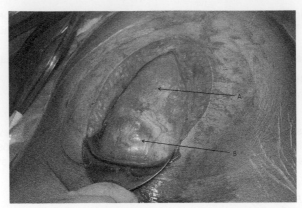

Fig. 4. Vertical skin incision for a suspected placenta accreta allowing access to upper uterus. (*A*) Normal myometrium (*B*) Placenta increta visible through thin myometrium and serosa. (*Photograph courtesy of* Dr Barbara Hoffman, Dallas, TX.)

Abnormal placentation can create aberrant vasculature and dilated vessels over the area of the placental insertion. In cases of placental accreta, the areas of placental invasion outside the uterus may also be affected by the abnormal blood supply. Care should be taken not to compromise the parasitic vasculature when entering the abdomen and exposing the uterus. With extensive placental invasion, profuse hemorrhage immediately develops with attempted placental delivery or if the placenta is incised during the hysterotomy. With uteroplacental blood flow at 700 to 900 mL/min near term, every minute of hemorrhage avoided is significant. If the placenta is in the lower uterine segment and especially in the setting of a percreta, fully developing the bladder flap and dissecting it around the placental invasion before hysterotomy can aid in prompt hemorrhage control and hysterectomy if necessary.[8] Depending on the blood supply, adhesive disease, and anatomy of the placental invasion, preparation of the bladder flap may also lead to bleeding, so the operator must use his or her judgment on the most hemostatic approach. In addition to preparing the bladder flap and avoiding damage to dilated vasculature, making the hysterotomy well away from the placenta will further avoid massive hemorrhage (**Fig. 5**). A transfundal or even posterior uterine wall incision may be required depending on placental location.[56]

With suspected placenta accreta, the most conservative approach to avoid life-threatening hemorrhage is proceeding to planned hysterectomy with no attempt at placental delivery and the placenta left in situ (**Box 2**). After the delivery, the cord is ligated and cut, the placenta is not delivered, and the edges of the vertical incision are quickly reapproximated, with either 3 or 4 towel clips or with a mass running suture, for hemostasis. Ensure adequate uterine tone with pitocin or other uterotonics as needed. The tissue around the uterus and placenta tends to be edematous and friable. Further reduction in blood loss can be accomplished by careful dissection of the retroperitoneal space away from the uterine wall, which reduces tearing and avoids puncture of the uterine serosa over the placenta.[56,58] Quick hemostasis can be gained by the delayed ligation technique where round ligaments, utero-ovarian ligaments and tubes, and uterine vessels are doubly clamped and cut from their attachments before any ties are placed. The clamps are then replaced with suture ligatures, beginning with the last clamp placed. Delayed bleeding once the engorged vessels normalize can be avoided by using 2 Heaney clamps for the vascular uterine and adnexal pedicles with a simple suture replacing the proximal clamp and a Heaney transfixing suture replacing the distal.[58] This technique is used to hasten the control of

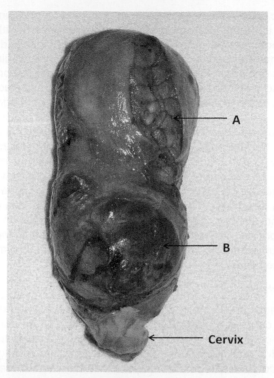

Fig. 5. Uterus removed with placenta in-situ and (*A*) hysterotomy made well above the (*B*) placenta. (*Photograph courtesy of* Dr Barbara Hoffman, Dallas, TX.)

major vessels and decrease blood loss but no clear advantage or improvement of outcomes has been shown in comparison to a traditional technique.[59]

When placental bladder invasion is suspected, the extent of invasion can be evaluated by cystotomy once the uterine blood supply is interrupted. If the trigone is not involved in the placental invasion, the involved portion of the bladder can be resected or left adherent to the uterus. In cases with extensive placental invasion into the bladder, the placenta can derive large amounts of its blood supply from collateral vessels of the bladder. Despite ligation of the uterine arteries, efforts to free an adherent bladder involved in a placenta percreta can often lead to severe hemorrhage and should be avoided.[60,61]

Box 2
Most conservative surgical approach

- Doral lithotomy position
- Vertical midline skin incision
- Dissect bladder flap before delivery
- Classical uterine incision away from the placenta
- No attempt at placenta removal
- Placenta left in situ
- Hysterectomy

A 2010 systemic review of emergent peripartum hysterectomy found approximately equal numbers of subtotal and total hysterectomies performed. With placental invasion, total hysterectomy was more common because of increased bleeding at the lower uterine segment or cervix but was associated with more vaginal cuff bleeding and increased risk of bladder injury.[62] The comparison did not find one method superior to the other so whether to perform a subtotal or total hysterectomy should be based on location of the placenta, level of invasion, and hemorrhage control.

With imaging modalities having only a 63% to 88% positive predictive value, when future fertility is desired and index of suspicion for placenta accreta is low, an initial attempt to deliver the placenta is reasonable. If the placenta separates or the diagnosis of accreta was not anticipated, a focal area of invasion or bleeding from the placental bed may be discovered after placental removal. If oversewing the placental bed is not adequate, successful treatment with uterine tamponade via a balloon or packing has been described.[63] A hemostatic square suturing technique to approximate posterior and anterior uterine walls, especially in areas with heavy bleeding, has also been reported. Of the 23 cases where the square suturing technique was described, all resumed normal menstrual function and 6 had confirmation of normal postpartum uterine cavities.[64]

Persistent Hemorrhage

Massive hemorrhage can lead to coagulopathy and tissue edema/friability can lead to bleeding not fully controlled after removal of the uterus. Diffuse nonarterial bleeding cannot always be controlled with surgical management, especially in cases of severe coagulopathy. Pelvic packing for controlling severe pelvic hemorrhage was described in the 1920s and continues to be a valid option that may permit time for correction of coagulopathy and hemodynamic stabilization. Various techniques have been described, most commonly using laparotomy sponges or gauze bandages, but the main goal is compression of bleeding tissues against the firm bones and fascia of the pelvis. Intraperitoneal placement of a large-gauge, closed system drain, such as a Jackson-Pratt drain, can be helpful to monitor for significant postoperative bleeding. Prophylactic broad-spectrum antibiotics should be used while the pack is in place.[65]

Uterine artery and hypogastric artery ligation are often mentioned in conjunction with severe postpartum hemorrhage. Eller and colleagues[66] found no advantage with bilateral hypogastric artery ligation but other authors report successful use of the technique.[67] The technique requires surgical experience in the retroperitoneum and visualization may be difficult with severe hemorrhage. Careful manipulation of the hypogastric artery must be performed lateral to medial and absorbable suture should be placed 3 cm distal to the bifurcation of the common iliac artery to avoid the posterior branch of the internal iliac artery. Possible complications include limb and/or tissue ischemia as well as hemorrhage if the iliac vein is compromised during dissection.[68]

Time-limited compression of the abdominal aorta below the level of the renal arteries can be a temporary intervention during massive postpartum hemorrhage, which allows for resuscitation with blood products and surgical hemostasis.[69,70]

Alternative Therapies

Alternative approaches to the management of placenta accreta have been reported whereby the placenta is left in situ and a hysterectomy is not performed. Most involve ligation of the umbilical cord close to the insertion site, either avoiding attempts at placental separation completely or minimizing the placental size with resection and retention of only the adherent placental segments, and closure of the hysterotomy without hysterectomy. Additional treatments used with alternative approaches included arterial ligation (such as bilateral hypogastric artery ligation), embolization with interventional radiology, administration of uterotonics, and/or methotrexate therapy. The placenta is either reabsorbed or removed at a later date with curettage and/or hysteroscopic resection.[71,72]

The 2010 French retrospective multicenter study included women over a 14-year period and reviewed 167 women treated with conservative management. Successful conservative treatment, defined as uterine preservation, was reported in 78%, but there was a 28% overall rate of infection, 11% incidence of delayed postpartum hemorrhage, and 6% occurrence of severe maternal morbidity to include sepsis, septic shock, and 1 maternal death (from complications secondary to methotrexate therapy).[72] Of the women successfully contacted for follow-up, 92% spontaneously resumed menstruation, 63% did not desire another pregnancy because of fear of placenta accreta recurrence, and 25% of them had subsequent spontaneous pregnancies.[73]

Conservative therapy obviously does not come without serious and genuine risks and should only be consider for patients with strong future fertility desires or in cases of severe invasion where full placental removal is not possible. If conservative treatment is entertained, a detailed discussion with the patient about the significant risk involved must be undertaken.

Methotrexate

Conflicting information has been reported about the use of methotrexate to aid in placental reabsorption. As methotrexate is a folate antagonist and decreases trophoblast activity, it has been suggested that administration will decrease placental vascularity and lead to placental necrosis and absorption. It is unknown whether the halting of trophoblastic cell division after delivery impedes this process.[74] The dosing of methotrexate that has been used is highly variable, ranging from one 50-mg intramuscular postpartum dose to a 50-mg dose injected into the umbilical vein at the time of cesarean section with a 50-mg intramuscular dose postoperatively within 4 days followed by weekly 50-mg intramuscular doses for up to 4 weeks.[74–77]

One maternal death has been reported secondary to methotrexate toxicity after injection into the umbilical vein. Common toxicities are nausea, vomiting, diarrhea, and mucosal ulcers, but numerous other side effects exist including leukopenia, anemia, gastrointestinal ulcerations, dose-related hepatotoxicity, and a rare hypersensitivity-like lung reaction.[78] Many patients treated conservatively and studied retrospectively did not receive methotrexate and placental absorption still occurred. In the 2010 French study, only 12% of patients received methotrexate. In addition to the 1 maternal death, cases of methotrexate failure have also been reported.[72,75] No high-quality evidence exists to support the use of methotrexate therapy with conservative management.

Postoperative Care

Patients undergoing peripartum hysterectomy, especially in the setting of massive blood loss and transfusion of large amounts of blood products, often require intensive care postoperatively. These patients are in danger of complications related to intraoperative hypotension, anemia, continued coagulopathy, possible recurrent hemorrhage, and prolonged operative time. Respiratory, cardiac, renal, endocrine and other organ system dysfunction is common. Pulmonary edema, acute respiratory distress syndrome, renal failure requiring dialysis, acute tubular necrosis, and, with large transfusions, transfusion-related lung injury have all been reported.[49]

Patients should have close monitoring of their vital signs, strict inputs and outputs recorded with urine output being measured via an indwelling urinary catheter, centralized monitoring with assessment of peripheral oxygenation by pulse oximetry, and initial trending of electrolytes, complete blood counts, and coagulation studies to include fibrinogen. Correction of persistent severe anemia or coagulopathies with further blood products and treatment of electrolyte abnormalities is important for continued stabilization of the patient.

When patients require intensive care unit admission, the obstetric surgeon often cares for the patient in conjunction with a critical care specialist. It is imperative that the obstetrician continue to evaluate the patient for potential postoperative bleeding from the abdominal incision, vagina, and intra-abdominal or even a retroperitoneal source. The surgeon should have a low threshold for re-exploration and hemorrhage control when bleeding is suspected.[79] Urinary tract injury during cesarean hysterectomy for invasive placenta has been reported to be as high as 29%.[80] In the setting of persistent hematuria, low urine output with normovolemia, or anuria an unrecognized urologic injury should be considered.

Appropriate thromboprophylaxis based on the patient's individual risk factors and postpartum hypercoagulability state should also be initiated. Many will only need intermittent compression devices while on bed rest and early ambulation. The guidelines in the American College Obstetrics and Gynecology Practice Bulletin Number 84 should be referred to concerning this practice.[81]

SUMMARY

- The incidence of placenta accreta has risen 13-fold since the early 1900s and is directly related to the rising rate of cesarean delivery
- Women at highest risk for placenta accreta have a history of a prior cesarean delivery with the current pregnancy complicated by placenta previa as well as placental implantation over the prior uterine scar
- Management of placenta accreta at a tertiary care center and a multidisciplinary team approach improve patient outcomes
- Gray-scale ultrasound has 77% to 86% sensitivity and 96% to 98% specificity for diagnosis of placenta accreta
- MRI should only be used in ambiguous cases and gadolinium contrast should be avoided
- Delivery timing should be individualized but generally around 34 to 35 weeks estimated gestational age
- Acute normovolemic hemodilution, intraoperative cell salvage, whole blood use, and hemostatic resuscitation can all be tools to aid in treatment of predicted increased blood loss
- Interventional radiology techniques, such as hypogastric or aortic occlusion, may be used but likely do not alter overall major clinical outcomes
- Planned cesarean hysterectomy with no attempt at placental delivery is the treatment of choice
- Alternative approaches, such as leaving the placenta in situ without hysterectomy, have increased risks and should be reserved for individualized patients
- Patients should be monitored closely postoperatively and may require intensive care unit admission

REFERENCES

1. Irving F, Hertig A. A study of placenta accreta. Surg Gynecol Obstet 1937;64: 178–200.
2. Breen JL, Neubecker R, Gregori CA, et al. Placenta accreta, increta, and percreta. A survey of 40 cases. Obstet Gynecol 1977;49(1):43–7.

3. Read JA, Cotton DB, Miller FC. Placenta accreta: changing clinical aspects and outcome. Obstet Gynecol 1980;56(1):31–4.
4. Miller DA, Chollet JA, Goodwin TM. Clinical risk factors for placenta previa-placenta accreta. Am J Obstet Gynecol 1997;177(1):210–4.
5. Wu S, Kocherginsky M, Hibbard JU. Abnormal placentation: twenty-year analysis. Am J Obstet Gynecol 2005;192(5):1458–61.
6. MacDorman MF, Menacker F, Declercq E. Cesarean birth in the United States: epidemiology, trends, and outcomes. Clin Perinatol 2008;35(2):293–307, v.
7. Hamilton BE, Martin JA, Ventura SJ. Births: preliminary data for 2010. Natl Vital Stat Rep 2011;60(2):1–26.
8. Cunningham FG, Williams JW. Obstetrical hemorrhage. In: Cunningham FG, Leveno KJ, Bloom SL, et al, editors. William's obstetrics. 23rd edition. New York: McGraw-Hill, Medical; 2010. p. 776–80.
9. Silver RM, Landon MB, Rouse DJ, et al. Maternal morbidity associated with multiple repeat cesarean deliveries. Obstet Gynecol 2006;107(6):1226–32.
10. Al-Serehi A, Mhoyan A, Brown M, et al. Placenta accreta: an association with fibroids and Asherman syndrome. J Ultrasound Med 2008;27(11):1623–8.
11. Sharp HT. Endometrial ablation: postoperative complications. Am J Obstet Gynecol 2012;207(4):242–7.
12. Pron G, Mocarski E, Bennett J, et al. Pregnancy after uterine artery embolization for leiomyomata: the Ontario multicenter trial. Obstet Gynecol 2005;105(1):67–76.
13. Lim PS, Greenberg M, Edelson MI, et al. Utility of ultrasound and MRI in prenatal diagnosis of placenta accreta: a pilot study. AJR Am J Roentgenol 2011;197(6): 1506–13.
14. Chou MM, Ho ES, Lee YH. Prenatal diagnosis of placenta previa accreta by transabdominal color Doppler ultrasound. Ultrasound Obstet Gynecol 2000;15(1):28–35.
15. Comstock CH, Love JJ Jr, Bronsteen RA, et al. Sonographic detection of placenta accreta in the second and third trimesters of pregnancy. Am J Obstet Gynecol 2004;190(4):1135–40.
16. Warshak CR, Eskander R, Hull AD, et al. Accuracy of ultrasonography and magnetic resonance imaging in the diagnosis of placenta accreta. Obstet Gynecol 2006;108(3 Pt 1):573–81.
17. Shih JC, Palacios Jaraquemada JM, Su YN, et al. Role of three-dimensional power Doppler in the antenatal diagnosis of placenta accreta: comparison with gray-scale and color Doppler techniques. Ultrasound Obstet Gynecol 2009; 33(2):193–203.
18. Twickler DM, Lucas MJ, Balis AB, et al. Color flow mapping for myometrial invasion in women with a prior cesarean delivery. J Matern Fetal Med 2000;9(6): 330–5.
19. Wong HS, Cheung YK, Williams E. Antenatal ultrasound assessment of placental/myometrial involvement in morbidly adherent placenta. Aust N Z J Obstet Gynaecol 2012;52(1):67–72.
20. Lax A, Prince MR, Mennitt KW, et al. The value of specific MRI features in the evaluation of suspected placental invasion. Magn Reson Imaging 2007;25(1):87–93.
21. Palacios Jaraquemada JM, Bruno CH. Magnetic resonance imaging in 300 cases of placenta accreta: surgical correlation of new findings. Acta Obstet Gynecol Scand 2005;84(8):716–24.
22. Briggs GG, Freeman RK, Yaffe SJ. Gadopentetate dimeglumine. In: Briggs GG, Freeman RK, Yaffe SJ, editors. Drugs in pregnancy and lactation: reference guide to fetal and neonatal risk. 8th edition. Philadelphia: Lippincott Williams & Wilkins; 2008. p. 804–5.

23. Wack C, Steger-Hartmann T, Mylecraine L, et al. Toxicological safety evaluation of gadobutrol. Invest Radiol 2012;47(11):611–23.
24. Webb JA, Thomsen HS, Morcos SK, et al. The use of iodinated and gadolinium contrast media during pregnancy and lactation. Eur Radiol 2005;15(6):1234–40.
25. Yang L, Krefting I, Gorovets A, et al. Nephrogenic systemic fibrosis and class labeling of gadolinium-based contrast agents by the food and drug administration. Radiology 2012;265(1):248–53.
26. Kanal E, Barkovich AJ, Bell C, et al. ACR guidance document for safe MR practices: 2007. AJR Am J Roentgenol 2007;188(6):1447–74.
27. Eller AG, Bennett MA, Sharshiner M, et al. Maternal morbidity in cases of placenta accreta managed by a multidisciplinary care team compared with standard obstetric care. Obstet Gynecol 2011;117(2 Pt 1):331–7.
28. Pacheco LD, Gei AF. Controversies in the management of placenta accreta. Obstet Gynecol Clin North Am 2011;38(2):313–22, xi.
29. Imdad A, Bhutta ZA. Routine iron/folate supplementation during pregnancy: effect on maternal anaemia and birth outcomes. Paediatr Perinat Epidemiol 2012;26(Suppl 1):168–77.
30. Krafft A, Bencaiova G, Breymann C. Selective use of recombinant human erythropoietin in pregnant patients with severe anemia or nonresponsive to iron sucrose alone. Fetal Diagn Ther 2009;25(2):239–45.
31. Harris SA, Payne G Jr, Putman JM. Erythropoietin treatment of erythropoietin-deficient anemia without renal disease during pregnancy. Obstet Gynecol 1996;87(5 Pt 2):812–4.
32. Effectiveness of perioperative recombinant human erythropoietin in elective hip replacement. Canadian Orthopedic Perioperative Erythropoietin Study Group. Lancet 1993;341(8855):1227–32.
33. Cazzola M, Mercuriali F, Brugnara C. Use of recombinant human erythropoietin outside the setting of uremia. Blood 1997;89(12):4248–67.
34. Hudon L, Belfort MA, Broome DR. Diagnosis and management of placenta percreta: a review. Obstet Gynecol Surv 1998;53(8):509–17.
35. Briggs GG, Freeman RK, Yaffe SJ. Epoetin alfa. In: Briggs GG, Freeman RK, Yaffe SJ, editors. Drugs in pregnancy and lactation: reference guide to fetal and neonatal risk. 8th edition. Philadelphia: Lippincott Williams & Wilkins; 2008. p. 640–3.
36. Committee opinion no. 529: placenta accreta. Obstet Gynecol 2012;120(1):207–11.
37. Chestnut DH, Dewan DM, Redick LF, et al. Anesthetic management for obstetric hysterectomy: a multi-institutional study. Anesthesiology 1989;70(4):607–10.
38. Stafford IA, Dashe JS, Shivvers SA, et al. Ultrasonographic cervical length and risk of hemorrhage in pregnancies with placenta previa. Obstet Gynecol 2010;116(3):595–600.
39. Robinson BK, Grobman WA. Effectiveness of timing strategies for delivery of individuals with placenta previa and accreta. Obstet Gynecol 2010;116(4):835–42.
40. Spong CY, Mercer BM, D'Alton M, et al. Timing of indicated late-preterm and early-term birth. Obstet Gynecol 2011;118(2 Pt 1):323–33.
41. Jolley JA, Nageotte MP, Wing DA, et al. Management of placenta accreta: a survey of Maternal-Fetal Medicine practitioners. J Matern Fetal Neonatal Med 2012;25(6):756–60.
42. Lilker SJ, Meyer RA, Downey KN, et al. Anesthetic considerations for placenta accreta. Int J Obstet Anesth 2011;20(4):288–92.

43. Kuczkowski KM. A review of current anesthetic concerns and concepts for cesarean hysterectomy. Curr Opin Obstet Gynecol 2011;23(6):401–7.
44. Kruskall MS, Leonard S, Klapholz H. Autologous blood donation during pregnancy: analysis of safety and blood use. Obstet Gynecol 1987;70(6):938–41.
45. Catling S. Blood conservation techniques in obstetrics: a UK perspective. Int J Obstet Anesth 2007;16(3):241–9.
46. Fong J, Gurewitsch ED, Kump L, et al. Clearance of fetal products and subsequent immunoreactivity of blood salvaged at cesarean delivery. Obstet Gynecol 1999;93(6):968–72.
47. Pacheco LD, Saade GR, Gei AF, et al. Cutting-edge advances in the medical management of obstetrical hemorrhage. Am J Obstet Gynecol 2011;205(6):526–32.
48. Cohen MJ. Towards hemostatic resuscitation: the changing understanding of acute traumatic biology, massive bleeding, and damage-control resuscitation. Surg Clin North Am 2012;92(4):877–91, viii.
49. Alexander JM, Sarode R, McIntire DD, et al. Whole blood in the management of hypovolemia due to obstetric hemorrhage. Obstet Gynecol 2009;113(6):1320–6.
50. Tan CH, Tay KH, Sheah K, et al. Perioperative endovascular internal iliac artery occlusion balloon placement in management of placenta accreta. AJR Am J Roentgenol 2007;189(5):1158–63.
51. Bodner LJ, Nosher JL, Gribbin C, et al. Balloon-assisted occlusion of the internal iliac arteries in patients with placenta accreta/percreta. Cardiovasc Intervent Radiol 2006;29(3):354–61.
52. Levine AB, Kuhlman K, Bonn J. Placenta accreta: comparison of cases managed with and without pelvic artery balloon catheters. J Matern Fetal Med 1999;8(4):173–6.
53. Bishop S, Butler K, Monaghan S, et al. Multiple complications following the use of prophylactic internal iliac artery balloon catheterisation in a patient with placenta percreta. Int J Obstet Anesth 2011;20(1):70–3.
54. Panici PB, Anceschi M, Borgia ML, et al. Intraoperative aorta balloon occlusion: fertility preservation in patients with placenta previa accreta/increta. J Matern Fetal Neonatal Med 2012;25(12):2512–6.
55. Sovik E, Stokkeland P, Storm BS, et al. The use of aortic occlusion balloon catheter without fluoroscopy for life-threatening post-partum haemorrhage. Acta Anaesthesiol Scand 2012;56(3):388–93.
56. Belfort MA. Placenta accreta. Am J Obstet Gynecol 2010;203(5):430–9.
57. Gilstrap LC, Cunningham FG, VanDorsten JP. Anatomy, incisions, and closures. In: Gilstrap LC III, Cunningham FG, VanDorsten JP, editors. Operative obstetrics. 2nd edition. New York: McGraw-Hill, Medical Publisher Division; 2002. p. 51–2.
58. Gilstrap LC, Cunningham FG, VanDorsten JP. Obstetric hysterectomy. In: Gilstrap LC III, Cunningham FG, VanDorsten JP, editors. Operative obstetrics. 2nd edition. New York: McGraw-Hill, Medical Publisher Division; 2002. p. 279–86.
59. Plauche WC, Gruich FG, Bourgeois MO. Hysterectomy at the time of cesarean section: analysis of 108 cases. Obstet Gynecol 1981;58(4):459–64.
60. Matsubara S, Ohkuchi A, Yashi M, et al. Opening the bladder for cesarean hysterectomy for placenta previa percreta with bladder invasion. J Obstet Gynaecol Res 2009;35(2):359–63.
61. Pelosi MA 3rd, Pelosi MA. Modified cesarean hysterectomy for placenta previa percreta with bladder invasion: retrovesical lower uterine segment bypass. Obstet Gynecol 1999;93(5 Pt 2):830–3.

62. Rossi AC, Lee RH, Chmait RH. Emergency postpartum hysterectomy for uncontrolled postpartum bleeding: a systematic review. Obstet Gynecol 2010;115(3): 637–44.

63. Vrachnis N, Iavazzo C, Salakos N, et al. Uterine tamponade balloon for the management of massive hemorrhage during cesarean section due to placenta previa/increta. Clin Exp Obstet Gynecol 2012;39(2):255–7.

64. Cho JH, Jun HS, Lee CN. Hemostatic suturing technique for uterine bleeding during cesarean delivery. Obstet Gynecol 2000;96(1):129–31.

65. Dildy GA, Scott JR, Saffer CS, et al. An effective pressure pack for severe pelvic hemorrhage. Obstet Gynecol 2006;108(5):1222–6.

66. Eller AG, Porter TF, Soisson P, et al. Optimal management strategies for placenta accreta. BJOG 2009;116(5):648–54.

67. Unal O, Kars B, Buyukbayrak EE, et al. The effectiveness of bilateral hypogastric artery ligation for obstetric hemorrhage in three different underlying conditions and its impact on future fertility. J Matern Fetal Neonatal Med 2011;24(10):1273–6.

68. Porreco RP, Stettler RW. Surgical remedies for postpartum hemorrhage. Clin Obstet Gynecol 2010;53(1):182–95.

69. Keogh J, Tsokos N. Aortic compression in massive postpartum haemorrhage–an old but lifesaving technique. Aust N Z J Obstet Gynaecol 1997;37(2):237–8.

70. Soltan MH, Sadek RR. Experience managing postpartum hemorrhage at Minia University Maternity Hospital, Egypt: no mortality using external aortic compression. J Obstet Gynaecol Res 2011;37(11):1557–63.

71. Bretelle F, Courbiere B, Mazouni C, et al. Management of placenta accreta: morbidity and outcome. Eur J Obstet Gynecol Reprod Biol 2007;133(1):34–9.

72. Sentilhes L, Ambroselli C, Kayem G, et al. Maternal outcome after conservative treatment of placenta accreta. Obstet Gynecol 2010;115(3):526–34.

73. Sentilhes L, Kayem G, Ambroselli C, et al. Fertility and pregnancy outcomes following conservative treatment for placenta accreta. Hum Reprod 2010;25(11): 2803–10.

74. Mussalli GM, Shah J, Berck DJ, et al. Placenta accreta and methotrexate therapy: three case reports. J Perinatol 2000;20(5):331–4.

75. Butt K, Gagnon A, Delisle MF. Failure of methotrexate and internal iliac balloon catheterization to manage placenta percreta. Obstet Gynecol 2002;99(6):981–2.

76. Lee PS, Bakelaar R, Fitpatrick CB, et al. Medical and surgical treatment of placenta percreta to optimize bladder preservation. Obstet Gynecol 2008;112(2 Pt 2):421–4.

77. Morken NH, Kahn JA. Placenta accreta and methotrexate treatment. Acta Obstet Gynecol Scand 2006;85(2):248–50.

78. Furst DE, Ulrich RW, Prakash S. Chapter 36. Nonsteroidal anti-inflammatory drugs, disease-modifying antirheumatic drugs, nonopioid analgesics, drugs used in Gout. In: Katzung BG, Masters SB, Trevor AJ, editors. Basic & clinical pharmacology. 12th edition. New York: McGraw-Hill; 2012. Available at: http://www.accessmedicine.com.foyer.swmed.edu/content.aspx?aID=55827134. Accessed November 7, 2012.

79. American College of Obstetricians, Gynecologists. ACOG Practice Bulletin No. 100: critical care in pregnancy. Obstet Gynecol 2009;113(2 Pt 1):443–50.

80. Tam Tam KB, Dozier J, Martin JN Jr. Approaches to reduce urinary tract injury during management of placenta accreta, increta, and percreta: a systematic review. J Matern Fetal Neonatal Med 2012;25(4):329–34.

81. Committee on Practice Bulletins–Gynecology ACoO, Gynecologists. ACOG Practice Bulletin No. 84: prevention of deep vein thrombosis and pulmonary embolism. Obstet Gynecol 2007;110(2 Pt 1):429–40.

Index

Note: Page numbers of article titles are in **boldface** type.

Printed and bound by CPI Group (UK) Ltd, Croydon, CR0 4YY

03/10/2024

01040441-0013